INTERMITTENT FASTING FOR WOMEN OVER 50

+ ATKINS DIET

2 Proven Strategies to Break Through a Weight Loss Plateau, Detox Your Body, Manage Inflammation & Blood Sugar

(+ Low-Carb Keto Friendly Recipes)

Nathalie Seaton

TABLE OF CONTENTS

BOOK #1: INTERMITTENT FASTING FOR WOMEN OVER 50

BOOK #2: ATKINS DIET FOR BUSY WOMEN

YOUR FREE GIFT

As a way of saying thanks for your purchase and to help you get the best results, we offer FREE bonuses to our readers:

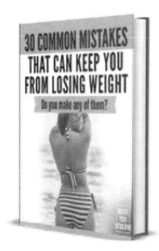 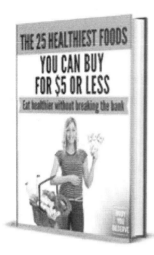 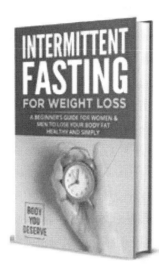 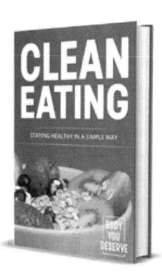

Free bonus #1: 30 Common mistakes that can keep you from losing weight.

Do you make any of them?

Free bonus #2: The 25 Healthiest Foods You Can Buy for $5 or Less.

Eat healthier without breaking the bank

Free bonus #3: Intermittent Fasting for Weight Loss.
A beginner's guide for women & men to lose your body fat healthy and simply

Free bonus #4: Clean Eating.

Staying healthy in a simple way

To get your bonuses, go to http://bit.ly/NathalieSeaton
Or scan with your camera

INTERMITTENT FASTING FOR WOMEN OVER 50

Balance Hormones and Reset Metabolism for Rapid Weight Loss: Look Better Than Ever and Detox Your Body with Autophagy and Anti-aging Secrets of Top Celebrities

Nathalie Seaton

INTRODUCTION

The best of all medicine is resting and fasting.

–Benjamin Franklin

If you've tried to lose weight, you've probably observed that it's difficult. Unanticipated health problems can bother you after age 50, preventing you from living the life you deserve. It's a lot more difficult than simply lowering your calorie intake and watching the pounds melt away. There are complexities beyond mere numbers—physical, emotional, and societal hurdles that a male-dominated health industry just does not address.

Men and women were made to be equal, but they are not the same—particularly when it comes to losing weight. In getting the bathroom scale to move, women face some unique problems. These difficulties include physical as well as emotional in nature. The causes include a combination of lifestyle and physiological issues that make losing a few pounds more difficult than when you were 30 or 40. (Not that it was easy then, either!) Women in their 50s experience everything from a slower metabolism to stress and sleep disorders that disrupt their diets. As they age and start living alone with their children moving out, women in this age group may be less active and fit, whether they notice it or not.

Female bodies differ from men's. Because they have lower lean muscle mass, they have lower resting metabolic rates than men. On a basic level, women burn fewer calories than males, even with the same amount of activity because of their smaller body size. In order to grow and nurture healthy kids, women's bodies have developed to hang on to fat cells better. As women age, their estrogen levels fall, and their metabolic rate decreases. They lose muscle and gain fat, particularly around the abdomen. Weight imbalances are also greatly affected by increasingly diverse eating habits. Because skipping meals and snacking are becoming common, distinguishing between traditional breakfast, lunch, and dinner meals has become more difficult. Diabetes, lipid profile, insulin sensitivity, and blood pressure are just a few of the cardiometabolic health factors that can be affected by such eating habits.

There are several other factors, such as genes that have a significant influence on how you age. However, you won't be able to do anything about it. On the other hand, there are some things that you can control, such as calorie restriction, or eating well but not too much. These are among the few things that have been demonstrated, at least in animals, to enhance life expectancy.

Diets have been trending for a tremendous amount of time. Diet pills were a trend in the 1990s. Besides, in the 1920s, a juicer in the house meant that you were aware of your well-being and health. Everyone has a different body structure and functionality, and we have to find a suitable diet plan for our bodies. But there aren't many diet plans suitable for all body types, age, and gender. Most nutritionists used to advise people to eat short meals regularly without skipping, but now they have shifted to a new mindset, which is clearly more effective. They present an alternative to restrictive diets called intermittent fasting, which includes occasional short-term fasting anywhere between 12 and 48 hours and is proven to provide many health benefits, especially for women over 50. Intermittent fasting, or intermittent energy restriction, is a collective term used to describe different meal intervals that revolve around voluntary fasting and non-fasting periods. It can have the same or even better effects as a calorie-restriction diet without aiming to actually reduce your calories. You receive calorie reduction as a consequence, and it helps to lose weight.

Intermittent fasting is one of the most popular health and fitness methods, which most people use to lose weight and improve their lifestyles. The method has also been proven to positively affect the brain that can help people live longer. People worldwide have practiced intervals of deliberate abstinence from foods and beverages (i.e., intermittent fasting) since ancient times. Fasting is an established custom that many religions and cultures throughout history have performed. Intermittent fasting is performed as a religious activity in many religions such as Christianity, Vrata in Hinduism, Jain & Buddhist fasting, and Ramadan in Islam. Religious fasting may just demand abstinence from certain foods or last for a brief length of time, with insignificant consequences.

Therapeutic intermittent fasts for the management of obesity have been studied since 1915, with growing interest in the medical world in the 1960s (Howard, 1975). The 5:2 diet, which we will explain later on, is a modern form of intermittent fasting that gained popularity in the United Kingdom in 2012 and has now spread to Australia (Barrett & Satpute, 2019). In short, intermittent fasting doesn't suggest what foods to eat but guides you when to eat them. You get to lose weight by enjoying your favorite foods! It's better defined as an eating style rather than a form of diet. One of the best things about intermittent fasting is that you don't have to count calories or make any particular dishes to stick to the routines. You can make anything at home or go outside for a meal. It's all about a little control and sticking to the regimen.

Intermittent Fasting (IF) has always been around in different types. Nonetheless, it was made popular in the year 2012 through a BBC broadcast by journalist Dr. Michael Mosley. Mosley appeared on TV film *Eat Fast, Live Longer* and published the book *The Fast Diet*, preceded by Kate Harrison's book *The 5:2 Diet,* which was derived from her experience, and then by Dr. Jason Fung's book in 2016, *The Obesity Code*. As testimonials of its success grew, IF built a consistent positive buzz.

In this book, you will discover how intermittent fasting can help you look better than ever and detox your body. Even celebrities like Jenifer Aniston, Kourtney Kardashian, Nikole Kidman, Halle Berry, and Jennifer Lopez swear that IF is their anti-aging secret. You will find more details about that in later chapters. You will also discover all about intermittent fasting and how different fasting methods affect us both mentally and physically. However, it is advisable to practice intermittent fasting under medical supervision if you have any kind of medical history or some conditions we will talk about in later chapters.

All in all, it will be up to you what fasting and eating periods you follow. Eating under a specific window will not only help you lose weight but also increase your metabolism, reduce the chances of chronic illness, and make you glow from within! All you have to do is respect the fasting windows, and you will have nothing to worry about.

I'm a passionate writer obsessed with achieving a balance between the pleasure of good food and an investment in what we have most precious: health. I'm constantly in search of the "perfect diet." However, I understand that the perfect diet for everyone does not really exist and that all eating methods have their advantages and disadvantages. I know that the best diet for you is the one you can stick to. Recently I learned so much about IF, and IF success stories from many women around me convinced me that IF really works. IF helped many women reach and maintain their goal weight and get rid of various health problems. This inspired me to create a book and help others get similar results, and I will do my best to provide simple, easy to follow, step-by-step instructions on how to do that.

So, are you eager to learn more about intermittent fasting? If you want to look and feel better, intermittent fasting will pleasantly surprise you. Let us get started immediately!

CHAPTER 1: INTERMITTENT FASTING BASICS

Fasting is the single greatest natural healing therapy. It is nature's ancient, universal 'remedy' for many problems.

–Elson Haas, M.D.

Intermittent Fasting is not a diet but an eating pattern made up of two periods: fasting and eating. One needs to develop a particular schedule to follow and be committed to. Without discipline, it can be a challenge to fast, especially in the initial days, due to changing eating patterns. Especially for a person switching from three helpings a day to say one, it may not be a walk in the park. However, it is worthwhile as there's a lot to gain from the practice.

Intermittent fasting is not a diet because it does not restrict a person from the foods they should eat. If you were eating bacon or beef every day, this does not stop because you start a fasting program. Most diets tend to limit a person on what they should eat, and that is why most individuals don't want to use diets for weight loss. IF, on the other hand, only determines when you eat the foods you are used to and love. But it doesn't tell you the type to love.

Most users of this method are aimed at certain health benefits or at losing weight, and you will learn more about the ways you can use it to shed unnecessary fat later on in the text. Meanwhile, here's a bit of information about how the process works: the body may exist in two states: fed and fasted. When you are either digesting or absorbing food, this is when your body is in a fed state. This commences once you ingest food and goes on for around five hours. Due to the high levels of insulin hormone at that time, it becomes a challenge for your body to burn fats, and afterwards leads to the post-absorptive condition. After food has been digested, absorbed, and stored, the postabsorptive state occurs. Skipping meals during the day puts your body in a postabsorptive condition. In this stage, the body must first use glycogen stores.

When you're in a fasted state, your body easily burns the fats since insulin levels go down. Most of the fats burnt during this stage were otherwise not accessible during the former stage. It is equally a rare state since it only comes about 24 hours after you have eaten your last meal; this is the basic idea behind weight loss using intermittent fasting. Your body is placed in a state wherein it is continuously burning fats. This state is almost impossible to get to when you are on your typical eating schedule.

Fasting affects several internal organs of the human body. This is an effect felt both in the molecular and cellular way. One example of a change in the body's operations involves the accessibility of fats. Using hormonal changes, your body makes the fats present for burning during a fast.

Again, IF helps you reduce the overall number of calories you take into the body because of a decreased number of helpings. Rather than eating breakfast, lunch, and dinner—as well as snacks throughout—intermittent fasting might force you to skip breakfast, lunch, or dinner. Therefore, IF primarily burns calories by making you eat less than your usual amount of food. This affects both sides of the equation, which is a positive thing.

In a period as short as five weeks, you can lose up to six percent of your overall weight by using this method. If you care about your health, you shouldn't aim to lose more. For example, the average weight for women aged 40 to 59 is 176.4 pounds. So a 6% weight decrease from 176 pounds equals roughly 10.5 pounds in 5 weeks. According to the Centers for Disease Control and Prevention, losing roughly 2 pounds in one week or about 8 pounds in a month is the golden figure for losing weight and keeping it off. That suggests that aiming for 4 to 8 pounds of weight loss per month is a healthy target on average. Just because you can lose a lot more weight, at least in the early months of a diet, doesn't indicate it's healthy or that the weight will remain off in the long run.

Insulin levels decline while human growth hormone (HGH) intensity rises when fasting. Your cells actively launch critical cellular repair mechanisms and alter the expression of genes (Kim &

Park, 2017). Intermittent fasting allows you to consume less food while somewhat increasing your metabolism. It's a powerful tool for losing weight plus visceral fat (West, 2016).

The Science Behind Intermittent Fasting

IF can be done in various ways, but all depend on the alternation of regular feeding and fasting periods. For example, you might consider eating at a specific time of the day and fasting the rest, eating from 10 am to 8 pm, and fasting from 8 to 10 the following day. You could also limit yourself to eating a day for eight hours, twice a week. Don't worry; later, you will find the eating plan that best suits your needs. For now, let's see what the process that activates the IF is. The body reduces its sugar stores and starts burning fat during the fasting hours; this moment is called the metabolic switch.

With IF, benefits are obtained when the body absorbs all the calories consumed during the previous meal and burns fat. When we feed, more nutritional energy is ingested than is immediately used. This excess energy is set aside by our body for later use, and in this, we are helped by insulin which is the main hormone associated with the storage of food energy.

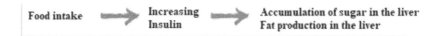

Insulin increases as we feed, helping to contain extra energy in two different forms: glucose and glycogen. Glucose units (sugar) can be linked together to form glycogen, which is then stored in the muscles or the liver. However, the storage capacity of carbohydrates is greatly reduced, and, if reached, excess glucose is transformed by the liver into fat. *De-novo Lipogenesis* is the name given to this mechanism (which simply means "making new fat"). Some of this newly produced fat is retained in the liver, but much of it is transported to other parts of the body. Although this is a rather complicated process, there are no limits to the number of fats that can be produced. Therefore, our body operates two important mechanisms of transforming excess food energy.

One is readily available but with minimal "storage" space (glycogen), while the other is more difficult to activate but has almost unlimited storage space (body fat).

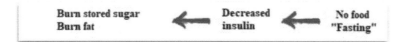

This whole process works the other way around when we don't feed. When we are fasting and no energy arrives in the form of food, insulin levels drop, signaling the body to start burning stored energy. Blood glucose decreases because the body must now take it from the depot to burn it and produce energy. Glycogen is the most readily available energy source, and it is broken down into glucose molecules to provide nutrition for other cells in the body. This process will provide enough energy to fuel most of the body's needs for 24–36 hours. After that, the body will have to tap into fat stores (and so break them down) to gain energy.

So, we and our bodies can be in two states: nourishment or fasting. In other words, we are either stockpiling food supplies (increasing supplies and gaining weight) or burning stored energy (decreasing supplies and losing weight). Still, if nutrition and fasting are balanced, there should be no net weight gain. If we start feeding the moment we wake up and don't stop until we go to sleep, we spend most of our time in the nourishment state. Therefore, we will begin to gain weight because we haven't given our bodies enough time to burn stored dietary fats. To regain balance or reduce weight, we can increase the average time used to burn food energy.

The Principles of Intermittent Fasting

If you eat every three hours, your body will continuously use incoming food resources, never managing to burn your body fat but rather accumulating it for when you eat less. Remember that if this happens, it means that you are neglecting the balance between the two states (nourishment and fasting) and neglecting the states in which your body can find itself; therefore, you neglect the IF.

Every routine or doctrine has a set of principles to govern the operation or process. Like any other doctrine, IF has principles that you need to observe when practicing. So, in this case, it is not a full fast, and as such, you are usually allowed to have a couple of helpings during the day. Here are other principles to take a look at:

You Plan Your Breaks from Eating

Intermittent fasting doesn't restrict you from eating. Instead, it dictates that you take breaks during set periods. In these breaks you take from eating, you are forbidden from taking any meal. Again, it is unlike the other fasting methods where a person avoids food every day for a week or month. Rather, in IF, you may opt to practice it once, twice, or more a week. The schedule depends on your motive and needs.

It is Well Researched

Nothing beats a method that is backed by scientific studies. Most of the contemporary and conventional weight loss methods people use lack a medical background; that is why they may either fail to work or work improperly. Intermittent fasting has gone through extensive research from scientists who have proven it as an effective tool for weight control. There have been substantial reports that illustrate the impact of this fasting approach.

Alternate Day Fasting

This principle of intermittent fasting involves interchanging the days that you eat more and fast less with the days that you eat less and fast more. Other models of this principle include eating as much as possible on a full day that you're not fasting and eating nothing on the day of a fast. In other words, you will be cycling your calories. The proportion of the fast day compared to the day you break the fast varies from one person to the other. In rare models, you will be fasting every day.

Restricted Eating

Instead of not eating at all, you can instead restrict your eating. So, you will not change what you eat or reduce it, but you will change your meal schedule. The timing, of course, is under individual preference and discretion. One well-known model of this principle is the 16:8 approach, which involves a fast of sixteen hours followed by an eating session of eight hours. We will concentrate on this and other models later in the text.

Whole Day Fasting

This is rare in intermittent fasting but is still done by some individuals. The advantage of this principle of intermittent fasting is that you will do it only once or twice for 24 hrs per month or per week instead of the others. This type of fasting has a lot of benefits compared to shorter fasting periods. I will cover that much more in detail in later chapters.

The Aim is to Burn Fats

The principle of fasting intermittently is to lose weight by reducing fats in the body. When you don't have food in your system, the body doesn't use sugar for energy. It burns fats and uses the result to boost your energy, reducing the overall fats levels in the body as your brain gets boosted. The human body is like a vehicle that needs fuel to operate. Food is the fuel that helps you move and perform different tasks. The typical procedure for energy formation when your body has food involves breaking down carbs into sugar. Your cells then use these sugars to produce energy used during different activities inside and outside the body. The excess glucose that the cells fail to use is transformed into fats and stored in the body.

When fasting, the body changes from glucose usage to fat usage for energy production. Once this happens, the IF magic is set into motion in relation to weight loss. Also, there's an even greater advantage when the body uses the fat stored in deposits for energy. According to science, when your body uses stored fats for energy in the place of glucose, fatty acids known as ketones arise in the bloodstream. Ketones help to preserve the brain and help it function better, in addition to causing weight loss. It also helps to deal with neurological disorders, besides boosting memory. Moreover, it supports the growth of new nerve cells inside the brain (McIntosh. 2020).

Studies show that when we eat food, particularly carbohydrates, the hormone insulin is released from the pancreas to deal with the bloodstream's glucose molecules. Glucose is either used at this fed stage to provide energy or stored as glycogen or fat. So, if you haven't eaten long and your bloodstream is low in glucose, a higher proportion of your burned calories will come from fat. In a few words, this means you'll be losing weight without doing any physical exercise. Of course, that's a dream for every woman coming true.

Science proved that we consume more of our fat during the fasting periods instead of eating times. But don't let the wording fool you. We are burning calories at any given time, and these calories come in different proportions from fats and glucose (carbs) (Fung, 2018). For instance, when I eat 2000 calories a day in 3 meals and skip one meal, I miss about 700 calories. When I eat 1300 calories and burn 2000 calories, I have a 700 calories deficit that will be burned from my body fat.

While it is important to keep your weight at a healthy level, it is equally important to do so in a manner that doesn't further damage your body. If you are looking at a particular diet to lose weight, be sure to do your research. Beware that one study on animal participants only does not constitute actual research. The brilliance of intermittent fasting is its simplicity. Some protocols and add-ons can be built on intermittent fasting, but the basic scientific principles always remain. It's a tried-and-tested concept, as evidenced by references to fasting in some of the most ancient texts in history. Many cultures and religions still hold on to the ancient fasting practices because they bring amazing benefits!

The capacity for storage of fat, in contrast to glucose, is unlimited. If you continue to take in food before burning off your glucose resources, your body will continue making and storing fat (Fung, 2018). When this is happening inside our body, what we experience outside is that feeling of a slowly expanding waistline, your body feeling flabbier than usual, and a general decline in how you feel about yourself.

When we burn fat, our body becomes leaner, and we lose weight. I still remember my third month into intermittent fasting when my husband told me I looked healthier and younger. That's the effect of burning fat healthily but steadily.

It is also important to mention that triglyceride levels in the blood are linked to cardiovascular disease. So, the more we can reduce these levels naturally, the lower our risk of developing heart-related diseases later in life. This is key for women over 50 as cardiovascular diseases are the leading cause of death in women in this age bracket. Intermittent fasting also allows the gastrointestinal (GI) tract to rest and repair itself, which reduces the possibility of cancers and other disorders of the GI tract.

It takes for the body to reach a stage where it starts to burn fat as fuel is different for everyone, but most research puts it at 24 hours. If there were to be no fatter deposits in your body—which would usually only happen after about 72 hours of zero caloric consumption—your body would start to break down protein for fuel. This process starts with your muscles and then moves to your organs. This is not a stage anyone wants to get to as you permanently damage your body by doing so. This process of muscle wastage is why people with severe eating disorders or starving people due to a lack of access to food appear worn, and their muscles appear stringy. The benefit of intermittent fasting is that you can access the benefits of fat burning while avoiding the point of muscle wastage. In women over 50, this is especially important as our bone and muscular systems need to remain as strong as possible.

Essentially, our body is always in one of two states: a fed state where it produces glucose or fat from food or a fasted state where we burn stored glucose and fat. We gain weight if we continuously eat and remain fed without ever burning off our glucose and fats stores. This is what makes intermittent fasting such a natural lifestyle. This is because our bodies are designed to occasionally be in a fasted state. By contrast, our body is not designed to be in a fed state constantly, so if we are snacking every two hours, our body will never burn off our energy stores, and it will always just use the incoming food as energy. Remember that all human beings on this planet belong to the species Homo sapiens, which evolved 300,000 years ago. Practically all animals fast when they are ill or can't find food, and humans are perfectly adapted to eat nothing for a few days easily. The average human can survive for 30-60 days without food (with the condition that he will have enough water). Looking from this perspective, one day without food is a trifle. The human body evolved to survive long periods without food, and it was uncommon and unnatural for our bodies to constantly eat from morning to night as we do in the last decades.

Another process that occurs as a result of fasting is autophagy. Autophagy is a natural process whereby the body breaks down damaged or diseased cells and uses cellular material to produce new, healthy cells. Fasting has been shown to increase the autophagy rate, increasing the benefits of autophagy. In addition, fasting places cells under mild stress, which is good for them as it increases their resilience. As a result, they are less likely to be damaged or become diseased.

The bulk of laboratory research to date regarding intermittent fasting has been done on animals, but human participants are becoming more common. Real-world results from intermittent fasting speak volumes, though. Unfortunately, it is generally difficult to get any human trials approved by the FDA (Food and Drug Administration), so significant animal subject trials need to be done before moving on to human trials. The difference where this is concerned with intermittent fasting is that human trials, albeit informal and undocumented, have been done for centuries with phenomenal results.

Scientists have discovered the many benefits of intermittent fasting when limiting caloric intake for one reason or another. With this technique, many features of the body can be modified for the better. The real question is not whether fasting can or not, but how it will help you and how often you should do it. This fasting style has been shown to lower blood pressure and increase HDL (high-density lipoprotein or "good" cholesterol levels). This can significantly help control diabetes and can also help you lose weight. In addition, studies on animals show that limiting their calorie consumption increases their lifespan by up to 30% (Gunnars, 2020).

Studies in humans have shown that IF lowers blood pressure, blood glucose, and insulin sensitivity. It is logical to think that fasting will increase the life span if passed for a long time with these tests. The same results can be achieved by cutting calories by 30% all the time. Still, it has been shown to cause depression and irritability. Fasting is a solution that comes instead of just reducing calories and benefits without depression or irritability (Che, et al., 2021).

Intermittent fasting works by eating food every other day too. The days you eat, you may end up eating almost double what you would eat otherwise. You still get equal calories, but you also get all the benefits. This will reduce your stress level and improve your overall health level. This type of fasting is a great way to achieve better fitness, live longer, and feel better all the time. Everyone still wonders what the next big secret of the food industry is. People want to burn fat and build muscle by investing as little as possible. They want everything, and sometimes it takes too much, at least in most programs.

Maintaining Protein Intake

When you're fasting, it's critical to keep your protein consumption up. Protein is required to form and repair tissues such as bones, muscle, and cartilage, the production of enzymes and hormones, and the maintenance of a healthy immune system. It also adds to the filling factor of meals. Some calories are consumed once you eat to aid in the digestion and absorption of food. TEF is a phrase used to describe the thermic effect of food. Despite the fact that not all sources agree on specific percentages, it is obvious that protein contains a stronger thermic effect of (20-30%) than carbs (5-10%) or fat (0-3%). If we use a 30% thermic effect on protein, this indicates that 100 calories from protein will only be converted into 70 usable calories (Land, 2018). Protein Promotes calories burned therefore raises calories expelled. High protein consumption tends to enhance metabolism because of high thermic impact and various other variables. It causes you to shed more calories all day, even when sleeping. High-protein meals do have a "metabolic edge" over lower-protein diets since they cause you to shed calories (Pesta & Samuel, 2014).

Protein works in a variety of ways to curb weight gain and appetite. This can result in an immediate calorie reduction. In comparison to reduced-fat foods, high protein meals not only offer a metabolic edge, but they also have such an "appetite edge," rendering it much simpler to lose weight. As much as protein consumption is kept high, that succeeds on a meal-by-meal approach and a consistent daily calorie decrease. Late-night eating is another important issue. Some people who are prone to gaining weight experience eating cravings at night and overeat as a result. Such calories are in addition to the nutrients they consume throughout the day. Protein, interestingly, it turns out, can have a significant impact on both appetites and the drive to eat late at night (Meixner, 2018).

Protein aids in the prevention of muscle loss as well as metabolic slowdowns. Fat loss isn't always the same as weight loss. Whenever you lose some weight, your muscle mass decreases too. Body fat, primarily subcutaneous (under the skin) or visceral fat, that's what you truly need to shed (especially around the vital organs). Most individuals do not want to lose muscle as a result of weight loss. An additional effect of reducing weight is that your metabolic rate slows down. That means you shed fewer calories after you lose weight compared to the way you were before (Mayo Clinic Staff, 2017).

Based on a study done by the American Dietetic Association, women over 50 need between 46 and 54 grams of protein daily. That's about 19% more than women ages 19 to 30. Why? Between the ages of 50 and 65, people naturally begin to experience a natural decline in muscle mass due to hormonal changes. To maintain muscle mass, adults aged 50 and up must eat sufficient protein—not less—to keep their muscles strong.

Why Start Intermittent Fasting Over 50?

As we grow older, our bodies change. We feel more tired, lose the strength to keep up with the daily challenges coming our way, and sometimes want to quit. In truth, most women have come to terms with the fact they have gained a couple of pounds over the years. They have convinced themselves this is inevitable. There is no way to escape weight gain, especially around the belly area and thighs. It is part of growing older, as you will hear people say. However, this is not entirely true. Yes, the body changes, and it is only natural. But this doesn't mean you need to give up on improving your health and looks. On the contrary, it means you must try a little harder to understand how your body will be working from now on. And once you do understand, you must adjust your lifestyle to better suit your needs.

There are different challenges in every age group, from birth until you reach 100 years of age and more. When you are younger, you focus more on performance and appearance. On the contrary, at the age of 50, you have shifted your mind, and now you care more about your health and wellness. The longevity effect is particularly appealing, as you are already experiencing the negative impacts of time on your body. Even if you are fit and active, you still lack the energy you used to have. You are craving for a change, which will affect you from within. This is the time to take charge of your life, aging only under your terms.

Through intermittent fasting, you can reverse the entire process of aging. Even if it sounds too good to be true, you have seen it work. There is proof of what nature can do to assist us in our goals. If you listen to your body and comply with its instructions, you will get impressive results. Science has got you covered. There has been extensive research, leading to concrete conclusions about how the body works. You now have all you need to kickstart your metabolism, reset your body, find your inner balance, and optimize your health. And it all lies under the concept of intermittent fasting.

Of course, it is fair to say not all women are meant to succeed in this type of fasting. It requires hard work, discipline, dedication to your end goal, and a long-term benefits approach. Maybe men are more naturally advantaged with discipline. However, you are a powerful woman, and you know that when you want something, you can get it! You cannot anticipate results to become visible right away. This is not the way intermittent fasting works, after all. Of course, you will notice dramatic changes in the way you look and feel. But you need to wait until the magic unfolds. Every cell of your body will improve through this process, so you need to wait and let it happen; sit back and feel your inner healing take place!

Intermittent fasting needs to be adjusted according to your age group and other factors. For example, women who are pregnant or have periods may practice only limited methods of intermittent fasting. They should do so very carefully because very long periods of fasting may impair fertility. Women over 50 have more freedom to choose from various methods of IF, and I will help you choose the best one according to your goals: to lose weight, reverse aging, improve health, or another goal….

Moreover, intermittent fasting for women over 50 is an invaluable ally in your struggle to reset your metabolism, increase strength, optimize health, detoxify your body, and feel better. By reducing inflammation, treating chronic health conditions which were once considered irreversible, regulating hormones, and increasing your energy, you are sure to experience a wonderful quality of life. Isn't this something to look forward to? When you appreciate the value of health and wellness, then you never stop trying. With intermittent fasting, it is in your hands to thrive.

In a nutshell, if you are a woman over 50 and you still want to try out intermittent fasting, kudos. You are one of the few brave and daring women, who have read about the outstanding health and weight loss benefits deriving from this dietary pattern, and want to put that theory to the test. There are specific things to consider, but you already know those things. Once you complete these slight adjustments and create a safe environment where you can fast and eat healthily day in and day out, you are on the right path.

Study carefully and do not lose hope or determination, with a minor slip up or with results that fall short of those you have anticipated at first. This is the time when you need to be stronger than ever. If you stick to the plan, you will eventually reap the benefits of this magnificent lifestyle. Your body will be grateful; your brain will be clearer than ever; your heart will appreciate what you are doing. Why would you ever settle for the aftermath of aging when you have the remedy? Undoubtedly, our bodies and our metabolic rate changes when we get to menopause. One of the most substantial modifications that ladies over 50 experience is that they have a slower metabolic process and gain weight. Fasting may be an unusual way to avoid this weight and turn around the gain.

Research studies have shown that this fasting pattern assists in controlling hunger, and even individuals who follow it regularly do not experience the same yearnings as others do. So, suppose you're over 50 and attempting to change your slower metabolic process. In that case, recurring fasting can help you stop consuming too much daily. Intermittent fasting may not be an exceptional idea for every solitary woman. In addition, anyone with a specific health condition (often tends to be hypoglycemic) needs to speak with a physician. However, this new dietary pattern benefits females who naturally store more fat in their bodies and could have a problem doing away with these fat deposits.

Your body also begins to establish some chronic conditions like high cholesterol and high blood pressure when you reach 50. Intermittent fasting has been exposed to reduce cholesterol and blood stress, even without a fantastic weight reduction offer. Suppose you've begun to observe your numbers enhancing at the doctor's work environment yearly. In that case, you may be able to bring them back down with fasting.

Menopause is one of the most complicated phases in a woman's life, when our bodies begin to change and important natural transitions occur that are too often negatively affected. At the same time, it is important to learn how to change our eating habits and eating patterns appropriately. In fact, it often happens that a woman is not ready for this new condition and experiences it with a feeling of defeat as an inevitable sign of time travel, and this feeling of prostration turns out to be too invasive and involves many aspects of one's stomach. It is, therefore, important to remain calm as soon as there are messages about the first signs of change in our human body, to ward off the onset of menopause for the right purpose, and to minimize the negative effects of suffering, especially in the early days. Even during this difficult transition, targeted nutrition can be very beneficial.

What Happens to the Body of a Menopausal Woman?

If a balanced diet has been carried out in life and there are no major weight fluctuations, this will undoubtedly be a factor that supports women going through menopause. Still, it is not sufficient to avoid the classic symptoms of menopause, which can be classified according to the period experienced. We can distinguish between the pre-menopausal phase, which lasts around 45 to 50 years, and is physiologically compatible with a drastic reduction in the production of the hormone estrogen (responsible for the menstrual cycle, which actually starts irregularly). This period is accompanied by a series of complex and highly subjective endocrine changes. Compare effectively: headache, depression, anxiety, and sleep disorders.

When someone enters actual menopause, estrogen hormone production decreases even more dramatically. The range of the symptoms widens, leading to large amounts of the hormone, for example, to a certain class called catecholamine adrenaline. The result of these changes is a dangerous heat wave, increased sweating, and the presence of tachycardia, which can be more or less severe. However, the changes also affect the female genital organs, with the volume of the breasts, uterus, and ovaries decreasing. The mucous membranes become less active, and vaginal dryness increases. There may also be changes in bone balance, with decreased calcium intake and increased mobilization at the expense of the skeletal system. Because of this, there is a lack of continuous bone formation, and conversely, erosion begins, which is a predisposition for osteoporosis.

Although menopause causes major changes that greatly alter a woman's body and soul, metabolism is one of the worst. In fact, during menopause, the absorption and accumulation of sugars and triglycerides change. It is easy to increase some clinical values such as cholesterol and triglycerides, leading to high blood pressure or arteriosclerosis. In addition, many women often complain of disturbing circulatory disorders and local edema, especially in the stomach. It also makes weight gain easier, even though you haven't changed your eating habits.

The Ideal Diet for Menopause

In cases where disorders related to the arrival of menopause become difficult to manage, drug or natural therapy under medical supervision may be necessary. The contribution given by a correct diet at this time can be considerable; given the profound variables that come into play, it is necessary to modify our food routine, both in order not to be surprised by all these changes and to adapt in the most natural way possible.

The problem of fat accumulation in the abdominal area is always caused by the drop in estrogen. In fact, estrogen is responsible for the classic hourglass shape of most women, which consists in depositing fat mainly on the hips, which begins to fail with menopause. As a result, we go from a gynoid condition to an android one, with an adipose increase localized on the belly. In addition, the metabolic rate of disposal is reduced; this means that, even if you do not change your diet and eat the same quantities of food as you always have, you could experience weight gain, which will be more marked in the presence of bad habits or irregular diet. Digestion is also slower, and intestinal function becomes more complicated. This further contributes to swelling and the occurrence of new food intolerances and digestive disorders. The distribution of nutrients must be different: reducing the number of carbohydrates (and choosing complex carbs over simple ones) helps avoid peaking insulin and maintain stable blood sugar.

Furthermore, it will be necessary to slightly increase the quantity of both animal and vegetable proteins; choose good fats, preferring seeds and extra virgin olive oil, and severely limit saturated fatty acids (those of animal origin such as lard, etc.). All this is to try to increase the proportion of antioxidants taken in, which will help counteract the effect of free radicals, whose concentration begins to increase during this period. It will be necessary to prefer foods rich in phytoestrogens, which will help to control the states of stress to which the body is subjected, and which will favor, at least in part, the overall estrogenic balance.

The phytoestrogens molecules are divided into three main groups, and the foods that contain them should never be missing on our tables:

- Isoflavones are present mainly in legumes such as soy and red clover.
- Lignans, including flax seeds and oily seeds in general, are particularly rich.
- Cumestani are found in sunflower seeds, beans, and sprouts.

Calcium supplementation will be necessary through cheeses such as parmesan; dairy products such as yogurt; egg yolk; some vegetables such as Brussels sprouts, broccoli, spinach, and asparagus; legumes; and dried fruits.

Excellent additional habits that will help to regain wellbeing include limiting sweets to sporadic occasions, thus drastically reducing sugars (for example, by giving up sugar in coffee and getting used to drinking it unsweetened). Change your alcohol consumption (avoiding spirits, liqueurs, and aperitif drinks) and choose only one glass of good wine when you are in company; this is because alcohol tends to increase visceral fat, which is precisely what is going to settle at your midsection. A dietary plan to follow can be useful to have a more precise indication of how to distribute the foods. Obviously, one's diet must be structured personally, based on specific metabolic needs and one's lifestyle.

Chapter Summary

- Intermittent fasting is when you alternate between periods of eating normally and not eating at all for 12 hours or more. It is a more effective method than simply reducing your calorie intake because it changes how your body processes food. Instead of storing the excess energy from food in fat cells, it creates ketones from fat cells, which are then burned to provide energy.

- When you're in a fasted state, your body uses its stored energy (fat) for fuel. When you stop eating and enter into a fasted state, your liver glycogen stores begin to empty. Once they're depleted, your body starts using fat as its primary fuel source instead of glucose because it doesn't have the glycogen stores to rely on any longer.

- If you're over the age of 50, then you may find that it's hard to diet and maintain a healthy weight. The older you get, the more your metabolism slows down. It may be difficult to maintain a diet, and there is a high likelihood of weight gain. Intermittent fasting can help because it's easier for the body to process food while it's not in use. Many other benefits, such as the reduced risk of heart disease, diabetes, and cancer, come with intermittent fasting.

- Fasting is a time-tested natural treatment that has been around for thousands of years. It is effective because it reduces insulin signaling, in turn reducing inflammation and allowing better hormonal balance. This can help reduce hot flashes, night sweats, bone loss, and other common symptoms of menopause.

The next chapter will dispel some of the most popular myths surrounding intermittent fasting.

CHAPTER 2: MYTHS ABOUT IF

Intermittent fasting is incredibly useful in aiding fat loss, preventing cancer, building muscle, and increasing resilience. Done correctly, it's one of the most painless high-impact ways to live longer.

–Dave Asprey, an American entrepreneur and author

Intermittent fasting has recently gotten a lot of press. Some women, however, remain suspicious about whether it is beneficial, effective, or even healthful. Whether you're thinking about intermittent fasting or already doing it, it's critical to understand the facts. If you have all the evidence, you will be able to fast appropriately—and if you fast appropriately, you'll have a better chance of experiencing the weight loss, consistent energy, and reduced hunger sensations that have made intermittent fasting so famous.

There seem to be several misunderstandings out there. Fasting myths are not based on reality; they are based on rumors, guesswork, and faith in ancient wisdom. Let's debunk some of the most popular myths about intermittent fasting so you can make more informed decisions about how to use it as a health improvement technique.

Myth #1: Intermittent fasting causes starvation in the body.

Intermittent fasting isn't starvation; it's a conscious food consumption gap over relatively brief periods for health and wellbeing. One popular misconception about intermittent fasting is that it pushes your body into starvation mode, causing your metabolism to slow down. When food is limited, like during times of famine or conflict, people starve unintentionally. Long-term calorie restriction can force the body to adapt to the lack of food and enter starvation mode, which indicates the body's metabolic rate is drastically reduced as a survival strategy. Intermittent fasting isn't the same as going hungry.

Intermittent fasting avoids starvation mode adaptation by alternating between consumption and restriction regularly. Fasting for a shorter time while alternating between fasting and feasting actually enhances metabolic rate. Fasting for up to around 48 hours has been shown in studies to increase metabolism by 4 to 14%.

Myth #2: Intermittent fasting causes muscle loss.

Malnutrition can cause muscle mass tissue to be lost. As a result, it appears reasonable to assume that skipping breakfast will cause muscle loss. On the other hand, fasting has been shown to help preserve muscle mass compared to typical portion control. It has been suggested that a person must fast for five days or more in a row until a large amount of muscle can be used as fuel. Fasting may help this phase by boosting autophagy or eliminating old proteins in favor of newer ones, making them less likely to be weakened. Fasting combined with strength training has been found in studies to increase efficiency and muscular growth. Fasting causes a rise in growth hormones, which could explain some of this (Keenan, et al., 2020).

The truth is just because you aren't eating regularly, especially protein, doesn't imply your body is going into "catabolic" mode, as many women believe. According to the hypothesis that the body requires a steady flow of proteins to heal, sustain, and generate muscle tissue, fasting breaks down muscle fibers for energy. Furthermore, a substantial amount of protein from the final meal before a 16-20 hour fast will almost certainly make proteins by the time you break the fast. Intermittent fasters frequently consume a substantial meal of slow-absorbing protein before starting their fast. Remember that prolonged fasting can lead to muscle failure because "de novo gluconeogenesis" (an adaptive mechanism that synthesizes glucose from non-carbohydrate carbon substrates) starts kicking in when muscle glycogen and amino acids are depleted. However, none of these scenarios are likely to occur in 16-20 hours for women who fast intermittently and eat a large, nutritious meal before fasting again.

Myth #3: Overeating is a result of fasting.

After a fasting period, you'll be hungry. Many women feel that this hunger will cause them to binge eat. The evidence, on the other hand, disproves this concern. Most fasting trials enable participants to eat as much as they like, a process called ad-libitum eating. They can eat everything they want and yet lose weight. Many intermittent fasting approaches, in fact, cause you to ingest fewer calories rather than more. You'll lose weight gradually without shutting down your metabolic processes, thanks to the reasonable calorie limit.

In multiple trials, intermittent fasting has been found to be a highly effective weight loss approach. Furthermore, there is no evidence that skipping breakfast leads to weight gain. It's not to say you won't gain weight if you binge and overeat during your snacking sessions—you will. Intermittent fasting is an efficient approach for weight reduction because it causes physiological changes in the body, such as a drop in insulin levels while raising metabolic rate, norepinephrine levels, and growth hormone concentrations. The main conclusion is that you lose weight by creating a calorie imbalance over time, in which you consume less energy and expend more. If you do the math backward, you'll end up with more weight (Petre, 2019).

Myth #4: Fasting for short periods of time lowers the metabolism but eating frequently speeds it up.

Taking smaller and more frequent meals does not significantly increase your metabolism or help with weight loss. Indeed, the overall quantity of calories you take is more important than the number of meals you consume. Without a doubt, your body expends calories digesting tiny, frequent meals. The scientific word for this is the thermic action of food (TEF). The TEF consumes about 10% of your entire calorie intake on average, which provides a minor metabolic boost. On the other hand, if you have multiple small meals throughout your day, it will be harder to control how much you eat, and you will likely eat many more calories than you expect.

According to new research, intermittent fasting speeds up your metabolism by lowering insulin levels and increasing blood levels of the human growth hormone and norepinephrine for short periods. These modifications may make it easier to burn fat and lose weight. Fasting each day for around 22 days did not decrease metabolic rate, but it did result in a 4% drop in fat mass, according to one study (West, 2016).

Myth #5: It is best for your health to eat three meals per day.

Some women feel that eating three meals a day plus snacks is best for their health and weight loss, but this is just not true. Fasting, on the other hand, provides numerous health benefits. The three-meal-a-day plus-snacks diet does not cause the physiological changes in the body that have been shown to enhance the miraculous autophagy mechanism (the process of cellular repair). Fasting for a short time triggers autophagy, which causes your cells to recycle old and defective proteins. Autophagy may aid in the prevention of aging, cancer, and neurological diseases such as Parkinson's and Alzheimer's. Indeed, several researchers suggest that frequent snacking or eating is harmful to your health and increases your risk of illness. As a result, intermittent fasting is very far from unhealthy, and it has a slew of advantages over regular eating patterns.

Myth #6: To grow muscle, you must consume protein every three hours.

More frequent protein consumption has been shown in studies not to affect muscle mass. It's a myth that you'll have to eat protein every few hours and consume 20 to 30 grams of protein with any meal or snack to grow muscle. Intermittent fasting can help women increase muscles and decrease weight. To grow muscles, you should eat enough total proteins before and right after the strength-training activities. Gaining muscle requires a weight-training regimen aimed toward muscle acquisition while fasting and consuming sufficient calories to sustain muscle growth. Your body easily absorbs more than 30 grams of protein with every meal. Protein does not have to be consumed every 2 to 3 hours.

Myth #7: The brain is harmed by intermittent fasting.

Blood sugar (also called glucose) is the brain's primary fuel, and it thrives on it. For a handful of reasons, however, eating carbs once every hour is unnecessary for brain health.

Non-carbohydrate sources of glucose are easily converted into glucose by your body. The brain uses ketones as an alternative energy source during fasting, eliminating the need to provide the mind with a continual supply of dietary glucose. You'll not only keep your mind working throughout those periods of fasting if you force your body to burn fat stores and run-on ketones sporadically, but you'll also boost cognition, strengthen neuron connections, and stave off dementia.

Myth #8: Intermittent fasting results in hazardous blood sugar reductions.

Intermittent fasting helps prevent (and even reverse) type 2 diabetes by stabilizing blood sugar levels. Your body is both a glucose storage and production machine. With strategic intermittent fasting, glucose levels usually stabilize, and the body undergoes significant changes and even reverses insulin-resistant disorders, such as diabetes, over time. Hypoglycemia (extremely low blood glucose) is only used as a precaution in patients who have already been diagnosed with diabetes and diabetics who are receiving insulin or oral glucose-lowering medications. In these cases, you must obtain authorization from your health care provider to follow an intermittent fast. If you're doing intermittent fasting, she'll need to keep an eye on you and monitor your blood sugar levels.

Myth #9: Intermittent fasting on a regular basis is too difficult.

Fasting regularly might be challenging. Nonetheless, most individuals agree that it is far more convenient than traditional diets. It doesn't require tiresome calorie counting (you either eat or don't), making it a much easier weight loss technique for many women.

Furthermore, unlike traditional dieting, your sacrifice reaps many benefits, including improved weight and health and fat loss. Furthermore, you are not bound by any food limitations during your eating windows. When you eat less often, you spend less time and effort thinking about food, food shopping, and preparing food. As a result, you can dedicate more time to your favorite activities.

***

Chapter Summary

- Though intermittent fasting has become one of the most interesting eating patterns to follow in recent years, it is still not without its myths and misconceptions. The chapter discussed some of these myths on intermittent fasting.

- IF does not cause starvation or muscle loss.

- The three-meals-a-day-plus-snacks diet does not cause the physiological changes in the body that have been shown to enhance the miraculous autophagy mechanism

- The brain is not in any way harmed by intermittent fasting.

- You do not need to consume protein every few hours to grow your muscle.

- IF does not cause harmful blood sugar reductions.

In the next chapter, you will learn the different ways to do intermittent fasting and how to identify which is the right way for you, so you can get the most out of the practice.

CHAPTER 3: DIFFERENT WAYS TO DO IF

Intermittent fasting is a lifestyle. It isn't something that you start today and then end when you get to some arbitrary "goal weight." Something you start and then stop is a DIET. Intermittent fasting isn't a diet—as I said, it's a lifestyle.

–Gin Stephens

There are several intermittent fasting approaches, and determining which one is best for you is the first step toward success. This chapter will describe the various methods providing as much information as possible to guide you in an informed choice. However, during your journey, you may find that the chosen methodology is not the most suitable for you. Listening to your body is the most important thing; you are always in time to change your approach, and there is no shame in doing so. It doesn't always make sense to grit your teeth and evaluate how your body adapts to the new lifestyle. Especially for the most inexperienced, choosing a softer initial approach and a more forgiving eating pattern the best way to start with the right foot.

The 12:12 Method

12:12 intermittent fasting is a type of time-restricted fasting. It is the easiest of all the fasting patterns. Everybody should be able to do a 12 hour fast. It is very much recommended for beginners who are used to frequently eating at regular intervals.

As the name suggests, the 12:12 intermittent fasting pattern follows 12 hours of fasts followed by 12 hours of eating.

This fasting pattern is deemed easiest because if you have your dinner by 7 PM, you can have your breakfast at 7 AM. Between the two meals, of those 12 hours, you will be sleeping for a minimum of seven to nine. Three hours of waking time during the fasting period are easily manageable.

You may divide the waking time between the night and the next morning or complete the whole three hours at night after dinner and eat your breakfast first thing in the morning.

The intermittent fast does not restrict any foods, but if you are combining intermittent fasting with a low carb or another diet, you need to take care of the foods allowed or restricted as per those diet plans. Also, when combining two eating patterns, start with one, let your body get accustomed to that pattern, and then slowly introduce the other form. This is necessary to save your body from shock and prevent it from going into the 'fight or flight mode.'

This is how your schedule will appear when following this fasting method every day.

12:12 SCHEDULE

	DAY 1	DAY 2	DAY 3	DAY 4	DAY 5	DAY 6	DAY 7
MIDNIGHT	FAST	FAST	FAST	FAST	FAST	FAST	FAST
8 AM	First Meal at 8 AM	First Meal at 8 AM	First Meal at 8 AM	First Meal at 8 AM	First Meal at 8 AM	First Meal at 8 AM	First Meal at 8 AM
8 PM	Last Meal by 8 PM	Last Meal by 8 PM	Last Meal by 8 PM	Last Meal by 8 PM	Last Meal by 8 PM	Last Meal by 8 PM	Last Meal by 8 PM
MIDNIGHT	FAST	FAST	FAST	FAST	FAST	FAST	FAST

Advantages

- **A good option for beginners.** It's simple, easy to follow no matter what your lifestyle is like, and doesn't require you to change your eating habits drastically.
- It enables you to **break from the habit of binge eating** and stop snacking at midnight mindlessly.

- It helps in **clearing inflammation** and getting rid of damaged cells, thereby preventing cancer while also promoting healthy gut microbes. Fasting at night gives the body a break from the constant digestion of food, stimulates cell regeneration that positively affects cancer, heart attacks, and dementia.

- While taking part in the 12:12 eating pattern, you're likely to **sleep better at night** and wake up refreshed in the morning.

Disadvantages

While this brief period without food may help to maintain weight and control blood sugar levels, it will not provide the total weight-loss and health benefits of other intermittent fasting methods.

Which celebrities swear by the 12:12 Intermittent Fasting method?

The 12:12 eating pattern is a sustainable, healthy diet that women in their 50s, 60s, and beyond are finding helpful in staying trim and looking great.

Jeniffer Aniston has been following the 12:12 fasting method to maintain her weight and general health. She has been a vegetarian and has followed a healthy diet. Her diet consists of many fresh fruits, vegetables, and nuts that help keep her blood sugar levels under control. Jeniffer claims the 12:12 fasting method has done wonders for her keeping her energy levels high and providing the energy she needs to stay fit, trim, beautiful, and healthy in body and mind.

Jennifer Lopez is another advocate for the 12:12 fasting method for women over fifty. She has been following 12:12 fasting methods since 2005 and claims that it has changed her life for the better, giving her more energy, fewer stomach pains, healthier skin, and a general improvement in health overall. She is a celebrity that performs worldwide; she sings and dances on stage at top nightclubs in New York City and Miami nightclubs to millions of adoring fans at her concerts around the world.

Shania Twain, the country and western singer, has been following the 12:12 fasting method since 2005 after discovering it on a trip to Switzerland. She claims that this eating pattern helps her to maintain energy levels and allows her to keep up with her busy schedule of shows and concerts that have taken her all over the world, meeting millions of fans no matter where she performs. She claims that 12:12 fast keeps her healthy, strong, energetic, and fit.

Angelina Jolie believes in the benefits of women over 50 who have difficulty maintaining a healthy weight and leading a healthy lifestyle. The famous actress has been following 12:12 fasting methods for several years now with great results. She claims that this eating pattern has helped her keep in shape and stay healthy for many years. She says she could not live without her eating pattern as she says it keeps her energetic, trim, young, and beautiful and is vital to maintaining a healthy life over 50 years old.

The 14:10 Method

This eating pattern requires you to eat all of your meals within a 10-hour window before fasting for 14 hours. For example, if your first meal is at 10:00 AM, you must complete your last feed by 8:00 PM. This approach is similar to the 12:12 method; however, it requires a 14-hour fast instead of 12.

If you choose to eat from 10 AM to 8 PM, this is how your schedule will appear.

14:10 SCHEDULE

	DAY 1	DAY 2	DAY 3	DAY 4	DAY 5	DAY 6	DAY 7
MIDNIGHT	FAST	FAST	FAST	FAST	FAST	FAST	FAST
10 AM	First Meal at 10 AM	First Meal at 10 AM	First Meal at 10 AM	First Meal at 10 AM	First Meal at 10 AM	First Meal at 10 AM	First Meal at 10 AM
8 PM	Last Meal by 8 PM	Last Meal by 8 PM	Last Meal by 8 PM	Last Meal by 8 PM	Last Meal by 8 PM	Last Meal by 8 PM	Last Meal by 8 PM
MIDNIGHT	FAST	FAST	FAST	FAST	FAST	FAST	FAST

Advantages

- **Mood improvement.** When you start the 14:10 eating pattern, your brain will release endorphins that are commonly called "the happy hormones." This means that your mood will improve, and you'll be able to deal with everyday stress and anxiety much more easily. In addition to this, while taking part in the 14:10 eating pattern, it's common for people to sleep better at night and wake up refreshed in the morning.

- **Reduces inflammation,** which is often the critical source of chronic diseases like diabetes, heart problems, and cancer.

- **Better digestion.** Studies have shown that fasters feel lighter and have a more regular bowel movement when they're on the 14:10 eating pattern. This is because the body has more time to focus on improving its digestive processes. People who have digestive issues such as bloating, heartburn, or acid reflux often notice a considerable improvement after taking part in this eating pattern.

- **Healthier skin.** Most people have heard about the other amazing health benefits of the 14:10 eating pattern, but some are not aware that it's also great for their skin. Your body will produce more collagen and elastin which will help you maintain your youthful appearance.

Disadvantages

When it comes to weight reduction, it may be less successful than longer fasting periods, like the 16:8 technique, and it may be difficult for certain people to create a calorie deficit with this method.

Here is what stars are saying about the 14:10 fasting method.

To find out what all the buzz is about and why so many women are trying this eating pattern, follow these celebrity women over 50 who are doing the 14:10 fasting method. See what they have to say about the benefits and how they feel after doing it.

Laila Ali, the daughter of boxing legend Muhammad Ali, is a retired professional boxer and mother. She has been fasting 14:10 and credits her success to it. She says she enjoys the benefits of the fast even more than the benefits from her workout.

Cindy Crawford, one of the most popular American supermodels, has been a vegetarian for years, and she says that the 14:10 fasting method makes her feel 'clean.' The famous actress is also a member of the 14.10 fasting method and claims that she never has to worry about her figure or weight.

Jane Fonda is a famous American actress and fitness guru. She started the 14:10 fasting method in Los Angeles but has adjusted it and finds it more convenient to fast for 15 hours. She claims her skin looks perfect, and she feels 'clean' when she fasts 14:10.

The 16:8 Method

The 16:8 intermittent fasting strategy is one of the most common types of fasting for weight loss. It's commonly referred to as time-restricted fasting, though some varieties differ slightly. In the 16:8 paradigm, a person fasts for 16 hours and eats inside an 8-hour window. Some people miss breakfast as part of the 16-hour timeframe. So, for example, you could eat between 12 PM and 8 PM.

Some folks, on the other hand, prefer to skip dinner. With this, you may limit your eating window to 7 AM and 3 PM per day.

For this fasting plan, you may still eat the major three meals a day. Mealtimes can be customized, such as breakfast at 10:00 AM, lunch at 2:00 PM, and dinner at 5:30 PM. A person can finish eating their meal by 6:00 PM, completing all food consumption within the 8-hour window of 10 AM to 6 PM.

Fasting restricts calorie-containing liquids and food consumption to an 8-hour window per day. It entails abstaining from food for the remaining 16 hours of each day. Unlike other diet programs, which might impose stringent restrictions and regulations, the 16/8 procedure is more adaptable and based on the time-restricted feeding (TRF) strategy.

By limiting the number of hours one can eat during the day, this fasting strategy may help one lose weight and lower blood pressure. When combined with physical exercise, research indicated that the 16/8 approach helped individuals lose body fat and retain muscle mass. A more recent study found that the 16/8 technique did not impair muscle growth in women who exercised aerobically (Moro et al., 2016). This strategy is frequently used for body recomposition (burning fat and developing muscle); in this instance, it is recommended to undertake your resistance training at the end of the fasting window to maximize fasting advantages (burning fat and encouraging growth hormone secretion/building muscle).

While the 16/8 strategy can easily fit into any lifestyle, some people may find it difficult to forgo eating for 16 hours straight. Furthermore, consuming junk food or too many snacks during the 8-hour window can undermine the potential benefits of 16/8 intermittent fasting. To maximize the health benefits of intermittent fasting, consume a nutritious, balanced diet rich in fresh vegetables, fruits, whole grains, lean protein, and healthy fats.

A balanced diet is recommended for intermittent fasting to be most successful. This holds true not only for the 16:8 strategy but for all of the strategies outlined in this chapter.

It is critical to balance each meal with a wide variety of foods for the greatest results:

- Fruits such as apples, bananas, berries, oranges, peaches, pears, and so on.
- Olive oil, avocados, and coconut oil are all good sources of healthy fats.
- Protein sources include meat, chicken, fish, beans, eggs, nuts, seeds, and so on.
- Vegetables such as broccoli, cauliflower, cucumbers, leafy greens, tomatoes, and so on.
- Whole grains, such as quinoa, rice, oats, barley, and buckwheat.

In addition, I recommend eliminating sugary or calorie-laden beverages. It is ideal to drink only water; however, unsweetened tea and coffee are also acceptable during fasting periods.

16:8 Intermittent fasting is probably the easiest approach to follow and can help you save money and time on food preparation each week. Furthermore, this strategy is not too taxing on the body and may be readily maintained even over long periods.

I recommend that beginners start with the 16:8 technique and progress to more difficult approaches only once their bodies have thoroughly adapted to this new way of life.

This image shows how your IF will appear if you use the 16:8 technique every day.

16:8 SCHEDULE

	DAY 1	DAY 2	DAY 3	DAY 4	DAY 5	DAY 6	DAY 7
MIDNIGHT	FAST	FAST	FAST	FAST	FAST	FAST	FAST
12 PM	First Meal at 12 PM	First Meal at 12 PM	First Meal at 12 PM	First Meal at 12 PM	First Meal at 12 PM	First Meal at 12 PM	First Meal at 12 PM
8 PM	Last Meal by 8 PM	Last Meal by 8 PM	Last Meal by 8 PM	Last Meal by 8 PM	Last Meal by 8 PM	Last Meal by 8 PM	Last Meal by 8 PM
MIDNIGHT	FAST	FAST	FAST	FAST	FAST	FAST	FAST

Advantages

The 16:8 method of intermittent fasting is a popular eating pattern because it is simple to follow, adaptable, and sustainable in the long term. It's also convenient because it can help you save time and money by reducing the amount of time and money you spend cooking and preparing food each week. In terms of health, this method of intermittent fasting has been linked to a slew of advantages, including:

- **Increased weight reduction.** Not only does limiting your consumption to a few hours each day help you burn calories throughout the day, but studies show that this method of fasting can also accelerate your metabolism and help you lose weight.

- **Improved blood sugar management.** This fasting method has been shown to reduce fasting insulin levels by up to 31 percent and blood sugar levels by 3–6 percent, potentially lowering your diabetes risk.

- **Prolonged life expectancy.** Though there is little proof in humans, certain animal studies have suggested that 16/8 fasting can help people live longer.

- It helps **cleanse the body** and provides resistance against lifestyle disorders like obesity, diabetes, inflammation, and such.

- 16:8 fasting satisfies **the three E's:** it's easy to do, enjoyable, and effective. Many individuals find it simple to skip breakfast since hunger is generally lower in the morning. The activities associated with this time of day keep their thoughts from thinking about food. Dinner may be enjoyed as a family activity.

Disadvantages

This method of intermittent fasting has a number of health benefits, but it also has certain negatives and may not be suitable for everyone.

- Some people may eat more than usual during eating periods to make up for hours spent fasting if they limit their intake to only eight hours per day. Then weight gain, digestive issues, and the development of poor eating habits are all possible outcomes.

- When you first start 16:8 intermittent fasting, you may experience short-term unpleasant side effects, including hunger, weakness, and exhaustion, but these usually fade once you get into a routine.

- The 16:8 ignores the calories in/calories out theory. Eating more calories than you're burning can lead to weight gain, regardless of when you're eating them.

- Fasting from evening until breakfast the following day demands avoiding after-dinner beverages and snacks. These lifestyle changes might be difficult.

- Compared to other fasting methods like the 20:4 method, the 16:8 fasting method is too short for autophagy to occur.

Which celebrities had great success with the 16:8 fasting method?

Sticking to a strict diet is not easy, but some women find that 16:8 fasting has helped them lose weight and shed negative feelings about themselves. As people age, it's easy to feel more self-conscious and body-negative as wrinkles form. Women celebrities over 50 who have been successful in their weight loss with the 16:8 method share how fasting allows them to regain control of their health and life.

Many people know that **Halle Berry** is the mother of a little girl named Nahla, but not many know that she has been practicing the 16:8 fasting eating pattern for a while now to stay fit and look young. She began this eating pattern when she was in her 40s, and it has worked wonders for her. As a result, her energy levels are higher than ever before, and she looks better now than when she was in her 30s.

Jennifer Aniston has also been practicing the 16:8 fasting eating pattern for quite a while now, and she is also one of the many women who look great at over 50. She achieved this look by following an eating pattern plan that provides 16 hours of fasting with an 8-hour feeding window. She incorporates healthy foods in her daily meals, usually low-fat and carbohydrate-rich foods. Her favorite food is fruit, especially green apples and kiwis, which help boost her energy levels throughout the day.

Since beginning the 16:8 fasting eating pattern, **Kim Kardashian** has definitely noticed a difference in her weight and the way she looks. She has stated that her clothes fit much better now, and she is healthier as well. This eating pattern plan allows her to eat healthy foods during the day, like nuts, seeds, and low-sugar fruits. Her favorite food that she eats on this eating pattern plan is watermelon because it keeps her full for a long time, and it keeps her hydrated.

Christina Aguilera has been using the 16:8 fasting eating pattern for a while now, and it is working wonders for her. As a result, she looks great and has more energy, especially after exercising one of her famous dance routines on stage during her gigs in Las Vegas, New York, or London. She also adds extra foods like almonds to the menu because they provide her with protein, and they keep her full throughout the day.

The 20:4 Method

Stepping things up a notch from the 14:10 and 16:8 methods, the 20:4 method is tough to master, for it is rather unforgiving. Some people call this eating pattern the "warrior method" too. Warriors almost always ate one meal per day. This one meal consisted of what they hunted or farmed. It also talks about old warriors like Spartans and Romans who used to remain on an empty stomach all through the day and eat in the evening. During daylight, they used to stroll around with 40 pounds of armor, build fortresses, and bear the hot sun of the Mediterranean, while having just a quick bite. They would have a huge supper around the evening, consisting of stews, meat, bread, and many other things.

People talk about this method of intermittent fasting as intense and highly restrictive. Still, they also say that the effects of living this method are almost unparalleled with all other tactics. For the 20:4/Warrior Diet method, you'll fast for 20 hours each day and squeeze all your meals, all your eating, and all your snacking into 4 hours. From my personal experience, I can conclude that it is quite simple to avoid eating for 20 hours, and it is not as hard as it sounds, especially if you're busy during your fasting window.

People who attempt the 20:4/Warrior Diet normally have two smaller meals or just one large meal and a few snacks during their 4-hour window to eat, and it is up to the individual which four hours of the day they devote to eating.

The trick for this method is to make sure you're not overeating or binging during those 4-hour windows to eat. It is all too easy to get hungry during the 20-hour fast and have that feeling then propel you into intense and unrealistic hunger or meal sizes after the fast period is over. Be careful if you try this method. If you're new to intermittent fasting, work your way up to this one gradually, and if you're working your way up already, only make the shift to 20:4 when you know you're ready. It would surely disappoint if all your progress with intermittent fasting got hijacked by one poorly thought-out goal with the 20:4/Warrior Diet method.

During that eating window, individuals are encouraged to consume a balanced diet that includes enough protein and healthy fats. They can also eat one large meal. Typically, the eating window occurs at night so people can snack throughout the evening, have a large meal, and then resume fasting. Because of the length of fasting during the 20:4/Warrior Diet, people should also consume a fairly hearty level of healthy fats. The human body needs fats for energy, vitamin absorption, development of cell membranes, making hormones that can regulate blood pressure and sugar levels, and many other processes in the body. What's more interesting is that you can also pair this fasting method with exercise, but it is not compulsory. You can perform some level of activity each day, whether it's walking, jogging, or even lifting weights. I would say half an hour of any exercise each day is a good start.

People on the 20:4/Warrior Diet tend to believe that humans are natural nocturnal eaters and that we are not meant to eat throughout the day. The belief is that eating this way follows our natural circadian rhythms, allowing our body to work optimally. The only people who should consider doing the Warrior Diet are those who have already had success with other forms of intermittent fasting and are used to it. Attempting to jump straight into the Warrior Diet can have serious repercussions for anyone who is not used to intermittent fasting. Even still, those who are used to it may find this particular style too extreme for them to maintain.

Advantages

- This eating pattern is arguably one of the most effective methods of **losing weight** because it entails a more severe calorie restriction and also you can pair your fasting with exercise or increased physical activity. This fact, coupled with the fact that it can be used temporarily without much preparation for speedy weight loss before important events, such as weddings or photoshoots, makes it even more attractive.

- It's also one of the **most researched** intermittent fasting methods (directly and indirectly). Some studies asserted that fasting for up to 20 hours per day could assist you in improving your blood sugar control, which is particularly beneficial if you have type 2 diabetes.

- The warrior diet helps **reduce inflammation**, which is often the critical source of chronic diseases like diabetes, heart problems, and cancer.

- The fast has been shown to help **detox the body** and regenerate cells by helping the body get rid of toxins and burning stored fat.

- **Brain health.** The Warrior eating plan is also getting more popular because of improvements noted in brain health. This method has been found to assist in regulating inflammatory pathways that affect brain function. Other studies demonstrated that fasting has a preventative effect on Alzheimer's disease (Francis, 2020). However, research on this aspect remains ongoing. More human studies are needed to make a conclusion on the importance of intermittent fasting on brain health.

Disadvantages

- It's not easy to follow for everyone. Our ancestors may have understandably gone for up to 20 hours without food. Still, it's hard to condition ourselves to follow that pattern in our current society and environment, which is utterly different from theirs.
- It may contribute to binge eating. As you can imagine, fasting the entire day can cause unimaginable hunger and feelings of deprivation—especially for women who have never fasted in any way. It's also common for fasters to experience obsessive thoughts about food during the entire fasting window.
- Especially at the beginning, you may experience side effects such as loss of focus, fatigue, brain fog, dizziness, stress, hormonal disruptions, and mood swings.
- Pregnant women, athletes, and underweight people are not recommended for this method.

Which celebrities swear by 20:4 intermittent fasting method?

Many women celebrities from all walks of life have adopted the warrior fast to improve their health and enhance their careers. Here are a few who swear by it for its many benefits!

Eva Longoria Parker is a proud mother of two amazing little girls. She says to "eat your fruit and veggies at every meal with plenty of water." She also says, "I love this fasting method because you are allowed to eat ALL that you like," referring to delicious fruits and vegetables such as avocados, bananas, berries, and mushrooms.

By following the 20:4 method , Eva lost 11 pounds, fired up her metabolism, and got her skin looking younger than it did years ago.

Tina Fey started following the 20:4 fasting method. It took her weight from 148 pounds to 136 pounds, and she lost 4 inches from her waist.

Since following the fasting/eating program, Fey has said she feels "more energetic and focused than ever before."

She also attributes her glowing skin to the 20:4 fast.

"I think the part I like best is that when I look in the mirror, I see a slimmer version of myself."

Michelle Obama started following the 20:4 fasting method in January 2012, and she broke the fast in June 2012.

She lost 10 pounds and improved her skin's appearance. She has also mentioned that it is possible to lose weight while on a fast, but this is not the only factor that will lead to weight loss.

"I still eat a lot of fruits and vegetables, turkey burgers, lean meats, and fish. But I've learned that my body works best when I take breaks from eating every few days. I'm getting up early and working out before the kids get up. I'm taking time each evening to relax, shut off my phone and go to sleep early. Because when I don't, I feel it."

The 5:2 Diet

This fasting routine has been included in the list despite the fact that, in reality, it isn't fast. It is more of a calorie-restrictive diet or fast mimicking diet. However, studies have shown that this fasting schedule brings a lot of results for women and doesn't affect their hormonal cycle at all.

The 5:2 diet, also known as the Fast Diet, is a calorie-limiting diet that follows a prescriptive program based on days of the week.

This method is particularly effective for very busy people who find it difficult to organize themselves with a fixed eating window during the week. The idea behind the 5:2 diet is to normally eat for five days a week and drastically reduce the calories ingested for the remaining two days.

5:2 can be considered a part-time diet that does not impose strict restrictions for most of the week, allowing us to eat chocolate, pasta, or any food we desire for five days. Obviously, to avoid nullifying the chances of success of this diet, the recommendation is to consume a normal number of calories during the week and avoid falling into the phenomenon of overeating.

During the two days of calories restriction, calorie intake should be limited to 500 calories for women. You should aim to consume around 2000 calories per day during the other five days. This means that you seek to consume 3000 calories less in an entire week. Your 500-calorie days will help regulate hunger and insulin levels, naturally reducing your appetite, making it easier to meet the 2000 calorie limit for five days of the week.

No restrictions are imposed on the type of food we want to consume; the important thing is not to exceed the number of calories indicated. Following this diet strictly, you can expect to lose around 1lb per week in terms of weight loss. Of course, this figure can vary based on how physically active you are and how much you eat.

This diet method is not particularly intensive for the body, and for this reason, you can also continue it for long periods or until you reach the ideal weight.

If you feel that your goals are too ambitious, you can decide to do two or more cycles to insert some breaks between them so as not to make the diet too stressful. The duration of the breaks can vary; I personally recommend a week so as not to lose the healthy habits you have built.

Scheduling your meals during a 5:2 diet is not strictly required, but it might help achieve better results. I suggest keeping your meals in 12 hours, avoiding late dinners between 7 AM and 7 PM. You can use a more strict time window if you look for faster results—i.e., from 7 AM to 3 PM. By eating earlier in the day and extending the overnight fast, you will significantly help your metabolism.

During your 500-calories days, you have to pay more attention to your diet, as it is very easy to reach and exceed 500 calories. Therefore, I suggest you focus on the following foods that usually guarantee a balanced calorie intake and allow you to create delicious recipes:

- Vegetables
- Fish
- Eggs
- Small portions of lean meat
- Soups

The easiest way to fit three meals into 500 calories is by eating a plant-based Mediterranean-style diet with plenty of fruits, vegetables, and legumes. Also, try to limit refined grains and avoid snacks during meals.

Regarding drinks, I recommend you drink only water, but herbal tea and black coffee can be consumed if you want something different.

5:2 SCHEDULE

DAY 1	DAY 2	DAY 3	DAY 4	DAY 5	DAY 6	DAY 7
EAT NORMALLY	FAST or Eat max. 500 calories (men 600 calories)	EAT NORMALLY	EAT NORMALLY	FAST or Eat max. 500 calories (men 600 calories)	EAT NORMALLY	EAT NORMALLY

Advantages

- The greatest benefit of this diet is that it's simple to follow for most people. This is especially important for women looking for an easy dietary approach to weight loss that works.

- This fasting protocol would also be great for you if you're not into dieting and counting calories often or every day of the week since you only have to do the counting twice per week.

Disadvantages

- You may have adverse effects such as irritation, hunger, or problems sleeping, as with any high-calorie restriction. Furthermore, for some individuals, five days of "regular" eating might be a steep slope in relation to food decisions. It is natural to want to treat oneself after a hard day's work, which may translate into consuming more unhealthy food than usual on non-fasting days.

- It is not convenient to restrict oneself to only 500 calories a day, even though it is just two days a week; you can feel sick or faint from eating very few calories. Moreover, counting your calorie intake is a big inconvenience too.

- It is known as a fast mimicking pattern. This is because although you are eating food, you are tricking your body into thinking it is fasting.

This is what top women celebrities are saying about the 5:2 fasting method

This eating pattern is the talk of the town right now because it promises countless benefits without requiring you to completely change your lifestyle. Celebrity women over 50 are among those who have taken up the challenge, and their success stories are worth paying attention to.

Jennifer Lopez is a famous Hollywood actress and singer. In the past, she has been open about her battles with weight. In an interview to promote her film, 'The Boy Next Door,' she shared that she feels comfortable with herself for the first time in about three years and has lost 40 pounds. In that interview, Jennifer Lopez revealed how to stay slim: 5:2 dieting method. "I have been exercising three times a week, and I follow intermittent fasting," Jennifer Lopez said. "On my fasting days, I drink lemon water with cayenne pepper, black coffee or tea with lemon, and hot water with apple cider vinegar or ginger. I also eat a slice of spelt bread with almond butter."

Beyoncé Knowles: "I've always been a big foodie, and since I'm a mom now, I just wanted to be more healthy. My doctor recommended I do intermittent fasting, so I started off with the 5:2 plan and have enjoyed it much more than other diets that fast or count calories. It's easy for me to stick with because I love to eat so much! The main thing is maintaining my weight, which has worked out great for my hormones and metabolism. This eating pattern has been amazing for me, and I've lost about twenty-four pounds in the first few months."

Jennifer Aniston is famous for eating small portions at every meal, but she found that doing so made her feel unsatisfied and hungry. She had tried many diets and other weight loss plans before the 5:2 plan and had failed with each one. Although she didn't struggle to lose weight, it was still a struggle to maintain her current weight. The 5:2 diet has changed that for Jennifer Aniston as she practices it several times a week. She doesn't count calories like most people, but she instead makes sure that she consumes a healthy balanced meal on her non-fast days and consumes only 1,200 calories on her fast days. Jennifer Aniston allows herself to eat whatever she wants for the other five days of the week so long as the portions are small.

One Meal a Day (OMAD)

The abbreviation OMAD refers to "one meal a day." Because that meal is usually eaten in an hour, OMAD may also be regarded as a 23-hour fast or 23:1 fasting. This is the most stringent kind of time-restricted eating method.

Advantages

The OMAD diet has been around for decades.

- In a study published in the International Journal of Obesity in 1984, researchers examined its most basic parameters; they found that a healthy OMAD diet helped overweight or obese women maintain or lose weight. To maximize its results, many experts suggest following the OMAD diet in conjunction with some sort of physical activity.

- Because it doesn't require you to count calories or adhere to certain meal patterns, the OMAD diet gives you the freedom to choose what and how much you eat. However, for best results, it is encouraged to eat healthier.

- Aside from being an effective weight loss diet, studies have shown that the OMAD diet can be helpful for people with diabetes and other health conditions.

- OMAD diet also ignites autophagy. The OMAD diet encourages cellular health, which helps you stay strong, energetic, and healthy. In addition, it can help you build muscle, lower cholesterol levels and strengthen your immune system.

Disadvantages

When you limit your calorie intake to 1 hour per day, it is difficult to receive most of the vitamins and calories you need to keep your metabolism from slowing down. Using this strategy regularly, you will get the best results if you keep track of your body fat % to ensure that you are shedding fat rather than muscle.

A pound of muscle is heavier than a pound of fat. Your body will store the former and burn it off during exercise to produce energy, whereas the latter will be deposited on your skin or bones. How can you track your progress and measure if you are losing fat or muscle?

Even if you have muscle mass, your body may still be putting on fat. The key is to take your body measurements and weight regularly to track the changes.

If you have a tape measure, check your weight and body circumference (i.e., chest, waist, hips, etc.) weekly. If your weight goes up a little, but your measurements stay the same or keep improving, you are losing fat. If your weight is up but your body measurements go down, you are losing fat and building muscle. If your weight is up and measurements are up, you are putting on fat.

This is what women celebrities are saying about the OMAD fasting method.

In recent years the popularity of this eating pattern has skyrocketed, with women celebrities like Madonna promoting it to help them lose weight. Some of the celebrities who have had a successful OMAD lifestyle include;

Sofia Vergara, 57, has been practicing the OMAD fasting method for the past 20 years to keep her body weight in check. She said that this type of fasting has helped her maintain a healthy weight while also keeping in shape and feeling energetic.

The Queen of Pop, **Madonna**, implemented the OMAD approach after her doctor told her to lose weight fast and keep it off. In 2017, she was 126 pounds. In January 2018, she was 122 pounds. The following March, she was down to 119. Being a vegetarian and an OMADer allows Madonna to lose weight with no negative effects on her health. Her cholesterol is fine, and she has maintained weight loss since then.

Eat-Stop-Eat

In following the Eat-Stop-Eat intermittent fasting program, also referred to as the 24-hour fast, you choose one or two nonconsecutive days per week during which you abstain entirely from eating for an entire 24-hour period. During the 24-hour fast, you can't consume any food except for calorie-free drinks. So, in effect, you're aiming for a complete break from food for 24 hours at a time.

Though doing so may seem counterintuitive, you can still eat something on each calendar day of the week. For example, you may generally eat until 6 PM on a Tuesday and then fast until 6 PM. on Wednesday, resuming regular eating at that time. According to Brad Pilon, the Canadian author who popularized this intermittent fasting plan in his book, Eat Stop Eat, if you can't make it the total 24 hours, 20 hours will also work. You can eat whatever you want 5 or 6 days a week. If you're only fasting once a week, this plan is ideal for keeping up or starting a daily exercise routine. Just make sure you get your physician's consent before beginning any exercise routine.

Your schedule may appear like this if you plan to choose this method.

EAT-STOP-EAT SCHEDULE

DAY 1	DAY 2	DAY 3	DAY 4	DAY 5	DAY 6	DAY 7
EAT NORMALLY	24-HOUR FAST	EAT NORMALLY	EAT NORMALLY	24-HOUR FAST	EAT NORMALLY	EAT NORMALLY

Advantages

- It's flexible and easier to follow compared to other more stringent fasting programs because you only fast for 24 hours at a time.
- Myriad health benefits include weight loss, increased fat burning, maintenance of muscle mass, and increased insulin sensitivity.
- It doesn't have food limits or any other restrictions.
- It doesn't promote calorie counting.

Disadvantages

- Refraining from food for an entire 24 hours can be difficult.
- There's a danger of overeating after the eating period begins.
- Fasting for 24 hours once or twice a week may not be sustainable over the long term.

Top women celebrities success stories with the Eat-Stop-Eat fasting method.

Many women celebrities over 50 have succeeded with the eat-stop-eat fasting program. They are living proof that you, too, can get the results you want.

Popular TV actress **Kristin Davis** uses eat-stop-eat to get back in shape. Kristin, who plays Charlotte in Sex and the City, revealed she puts her busy schedule at risk by fasting but can see the results. She said: "I am a big fan of fasting. I know it's not for everyone, but I'm a big believer in it and try to follow it as much as my schedule allows me to. I tend to want to eat the same thing every day, and cutting out those calories is really difficult. I find that when I fast, my body goes into conservation mode. It's like I'm on a rollercoaster, and it conserves everything, so you can lose weight."

Famous American TV personality **Oprah Winfrey** is one of the celebrities over 50 who use eat-stop-eat to lose weight. Oprah said she follows the diet religiously. She said: 'Eat-Stop-Eat is working for me. It's so fabulous to watch myself losing weight.

It might surprise some to find out that American model **Janice Dickinson** is one of the celebrities over 50 using the Eat-Stop-Eat diet plan to lose weight. Janice lost 60 lbs (27 kilos) by following the eat stop eat method. She said, "Eat-Stop-Eat was an easy way for me to incorporate fasting into my lifestyle because it didn't require me to give up any of my usual meals. I have lost 27 lbs and still have a lot more to go. I'm at my goal weight, and I'm feeling great."

Longer Periods of Fasting

Short fasting can reduce insulin levels and therefore help prevent insulin resistance. However, eliminating insulin resistance requires persistent low levels of insulin. Therefore, longer fasting periods may be needed.

The Risks and Benefits of Longer Fasts

The benefits of weight loss and lower insulin levels are almost immediate.

Some foods are better than others but all foods increase insulin production. If all foods increase insulin then the only way for us to lower it – is to completely abstain from food. When we're talking about fasting to break insulin resistance and lose weight – we're talking about IF from 24 to 36 hours.

Eating continuously is a recipe for weight gain. IF is a very effective way to deal with when to eat. In the end, the question is this: if you don't eat, will you lose weight? Yes, of course. So, there is no real doubt about its advocacy, it will work.

Shorted fasts are general done more frequently. Some people prefer a daily 16:8 fast. Longer fast are typically from 24 hors to 36 hours done 2-3 times per week. Longer fasting periods produce lower insulin levels, greater weight loss and greater blood sugar reduction in diabetics

Fung and Moore (2016) stress that if you feel ill during fasting, you should stop the fast. It is okay to feel hungry but not okay to feel ill.

Anyone on medication, especially diabetic medication, should talk to their doctor before fasting. Diabetic medication is prescribed based on your current diet. If a diabetic person stops eating, there is a risk for hypoglycemia, which can be very dangerous.

Symptoms of hypoglycemia include sweating, tremors, confusion, hunger, shakiness, and weakness. If hypoglycemia is not treated, it can lead to unconsciousness and even death.

24-Hour Fasts

During this fast, people do not eat from breakfast to breakfast or supper to supper. There are many advantages to a twenty-four-hour fast.

- Because one meal is eaten every day, medications that must be taken with food can still be taken normally.
- It is an easier regimen to follow. For example, a person can skip breakfast and lunch but still have dinner with their family.
- Nutrition is not an issue since food is still consumed every day.
- This regimen can be followed daily, although many people get good results by exercising the twenty-four-hour regimen two or three times a week.

Dr Jason Fung, an expert on intermittent fasting, advises people who exercise the twenty-four-hour fasts to not restrict calories after the fast is over. He recommends eating a low carbohydrate, high-fat meal composed of unprocessed foods (Fung, 2018).

36-Hour Fasts

For this fast a person does not eat for one entire day. The person may eat dinner on day one, nothing on day two, and then eat breakfast on day three.

Fung states that this fasting schedule works for those who suffer from type 2 diabetes. The longer the person has suffered from diabetes, the longer he or she will need to maintain this fasting schedule.

Once the diabetes is under control, a fasting schedule can help the person maintain insulin and weight levels.

It is essential that diabetics check their blood sugar two to four times a day while fasting.

So, "Should I fast for 48, 72, or even 90 hours?" There is no clear answer to that because it's important for you to listen to your body and figure out what is best for yourself.

With that said, the longest fasts recommended by medical professionals are 36 hours. So, even if you go longer than that without food and water, it would not be recommendable. Why? Because it can put your health in serious jeopardy.

Longer fasts than that may lead to health problems such as dehydration, electrolyte imbalances, muscle wasting, weakness and even death if you have a pre-existing medical condition.

After 36 hours of not eating or drinking anything but water and in some cases caffeine/organic coffee (or tea), many people have reported that their bodies just can't handle it anymore. A few people have reported feeling like they are starving (which means your body is actually starving). And, if you are experiencing that, then you should stop.

It's better to do a shorter fast for a day or two than it is to force yourself to go beyond your body's natural ability and do extensive fasting for days at a time.

***

Chapter Summary

- Before starting intermittent fasting and incorporating it into your lifestyle, you must know all the possibilities to choose the right one for you, your goals, your habits, and your body/personality type.

- Shorted fasts are generally done more frequently. Some people prefer a daily 16:8 fast.

- Longer fasts are typically from 24 hours to 36 hours done 2-3 times per week.

- In diabetics, longer fasting periods result in lower insulin levels, more weight loss, and lower blood sugar levels.

- Try different IF methods to find a method you can stick to.

In the next chapter, we'll take an in-depth look at the steps in your approach to fasting, which will help you optimize your path to weight loss—or improve your life in general!

CHAPTER 4: STEP-BY-STEP GUIDE TO STARTING IF

Fasting, by taking a completely different approach, is much easier to understand. It is so simple that it can be explained in two sentences: Eat nothing. Drink water, tea, coffee, or bone broth. That's it.

–Jason Fung

In the previous chapter, I did my best to explain the various intermittent fasting methods to give you an idea of the basic principles of this eating pattern. This chapter will detail how to organize an intermittent fasting eating pattern that leads you to the desired results.

Step #1: Set goals.

Setting goals is essential for starting any new routine, including intermittent fasting. When you're clear on your goals, it's easier to stay motivated and focused as you make the necessary changes in your life.

Think about what you want to achieve with intermittent fasting: weight loss? Improved blood sugar levels or cholesterol? More energy? Better sleep?

Write these goals down and refer to them often as you begin your fasting journey.

Jot down three goals you want to accomplish through intermittent fastings, like losing weight or improving energy levels. Write them in the present tense as if they have already happened ("I am"). Remind yourself that no matter how big or small a goal seems, everyone starts somewhere, and anything is possible with consistent effort. For example, "By January 31st, I want to lose 20 pounds." Try not to be too specific, so it doesn't create pressure on yourself but instead focuses more on what you want to accomplish.

Step #2: Choose your method.

Now that you know exactly what you're seeking from IF, the next step involves picking a suitable IF method that will help you achieve your goals.

In addition to your specific goals regarding IF, other factors also go into choosing an IF method that would yield the most benefits for you. These include the length of time you want to fast for, your daily routine, what field of work you're employed in and what a typical workday looks like for you, the specific climatic conditions prevailing in your part of the world, and how often you dine out with friends and family, to name a few.

Once you have chosen an IF method, though, remember that you're not stuck with it forever. It is entirely possible to transition from one type of IF to another if you find that your current regimen isn't working for you or if you think you've mastered the moderate forms of IF (consider the 16:8 method) and want to go pro and explore some relatively challenging routes such as the Alternate-Day fasting.

Besides, a person should give at least one month's serious go to any particular IF method before quitting or switching it up for good.

Step #3: Start with 12 hours of fasting.

Start with 12 hours of fasting and work your way up as your body gets used to it if you're a beginner. For example, if you finish eating at seven on Friday evening during weekdays, don't eat or drink anything until after seven o'clock on Saturday morning (a 12-hour fast). Once you get used to this schedule over a few weeks, try extending your daily fasting window by an hour. Then gradually increase both periods, always aiming for consistency rather than perfection!

You can slowly extend your fasting time as you get more comfortable. If it's working, don't change a thing!

Step #4: Keep an eye on your calories.

Now that you know what you want from IF and how you're going to approach it, the next step involves finding a way to figure out and manage your calories. This is important because if your top goal for IF is weight loss, then you need to consume fewer calories than you burn for energy, i.e., build a calorie deficit. While IF is naturally designed to create a calorie deficit when you're fasting, this can be quickly turned into a surplus if you're not mindful of the calories you consume during your eating windows.

Some people practicing IF are not concerned about counting and measuring their calories. Although keeping track of one's calorie consumption is important to a certain extent (even while fasting intermittently), these folks are of the opinion that their calorie consumption is automatically taken care of as a direct result of fasting intermittently. While this may work out well for someone who doesn't suffer from (or is prone to) an eating disorder such as anorexia, orthorexia, and binge eating, it can be detrimental for individuals whose eating disorders may be triggered by IF.

Keeping track of the number of calories you consume during IF is also important because even if certain methods of IF, such as Alternate-Day fasting, do allow for calorie consumption during fasting days, there is a limit to how much of these calories one can consume. Again, this restriction is meant to facilitate the benefits of IF, such as weight loss.

Besides, there is a popular opinion that as long as you consume just under 50 calories in the morning, you will be considered in the fasted state. This can be critical for those practicing the 16:8 method by having an early dinner and delayed breakfast in an attempt to reach a 16-hour milestone with their fasting. Such people can drink plain water or have a cup of black coffee (no added sugar!) without the risk of breaking their fast in the mornings.

But guess what? This also implies that you have to be mindful of the calories you consume to ensure that your IF regimen is not put to waste.

All of this leads to one conclusion only: whether you're fasting or feasting, you must keep an eye on your calorie consumption to achieve your goals with IF. At least in the beginning.

Nowadays, there are a variety of apps that can be used to track calorie intake. Some of the best ones include MyFitnessPal and Lose It!, which include a calorie counter, food diary, and exercise log.

As you get the hang of doing IF in any shape or form that you think best suits you and your situation, the focus on calorie intake will usually wind up fading into the background as IF and your new eating habits get ingrained into your schedule. You will find that you do not need to track the calories as much because you know the approximate amounts you consume daily. This is when the much-vaunted benefit of not needing to calorie count comes back straight into play, with a vengeance! Because you have more practice and have already established a fair routine and habit in your IF lifestyle, your daily caloric intake is more or less at your fingertips. Consequently, you end up not paying too much attention to that and can carry on with your daily stuff without worrying about the calorie count.

Step #5: Plan your meals.

Meal planning is critical when intermittent fasting. This way, you'll know exactly what to eat and when to eat it, so you don't have to worry about making last-minute decisions that could sabotage your diet plan.

When creating your meal plan, include plenty of healthy fats, protein, and complex carbohydrates. Here are some ideas for each category:

- **Healthy Fats:** olive oil, coconut oil, nuts (almonds, walnuts, pistachios), seeds (pumpkin seeds, sunflower seeds)
- **Protein:** chicken breast, salmon, shrimp, tofu, eggs

- **Complex Carbohydrates:** whole grain pasta, quinoa, brown rice, sweet potatoes, Ezekiel bread

It's also helpful to plan out your meals and snacks for the week, so you're not tempted to reach for unhealthy options when you get hungry.

It is advisable to plan your fasting windows when you sleep or are busy doing something for a longer time—that will help you avoid thinking about food when you should be not eating.

Step #6: Drink plenty of water.

Water is essential when fasting and helps flush toxins from the body. Ensure that you consume an adequate amount of water—at least eight glasses per day—throughout your fasting period. Herbal tea or black coffee are also allowed.

Step #7: Reward yourself along the way.

Although intermittent fasting should never be viewed as a punishment, it's okay—encouraged even—to reward yourself for sticking to your program. Maybe allow yourself a small snack or drink after completing a successful fast, or buy yourself something nice that you've been wanting. Just be sure to keep your rewards in check, and don't overdo it!

Chapter Summary

- Defining your goals when it comes to IF allows you to pick the most suitable IF method that will effectively take you closer to what you want.

- Building up a new habit should be started slowly and steadily. Starting a project on a shorter timeline can prevent you from getting worn out. So, if you don't feel like eating, fasting can be a good way to kick-start your day.

- Start slow, then gradually increase the duration of the fast as the body adapts to the new regime.

- Prepare your meals the day before your fast days; this helps you stay on track and reduces food waste.

- It is very important to constantly hydrate yourself. About two liters of water consumption in a day is necessary.

- It is critical to reward yourself on days when you can resume normal eating. A small reward can go a long way toward reminding yourself and your brain that what you're doing is worthwhile and should be recognized.

No matter how you plot your path for an intermittent fast, you need to understand what is good to eat and not to eat during your efforts. The next chapter will help guide you to make wise food choices on what to eat and what not to eat during your intermittent fasting.

CHAPTER 5: WHAT TO EAT

The basics of good nutrition can be summarized in these simple rules. Eat whole, unprocessed foods. Avoid sugar. Avoid refined grains. Eat a diet high in natural fats. Balance feeding with fasting!

–Jason Fung

IF is a lifestyle change, and to ensure your success with the practice, you might have to re-learn some of your eating habits. This chapter walks you through how to do this important task while fasting intermittently.

Although IF does not explicitly put any restrictions on what you should eat or avoid consuming altogether, it won't do harm to follow some general guidelines for eating nonetheless.

These recommendations are only meant to enhance the health benefits you might expect from following an IF regimen.

It is also recommended to have the assistance of a nutritionist to practice intermittent fasting, as this professional will be able to set up the best diet for you.

Intermittent fasting divides the routine into three parts: foods you can eat while fasting, foods to eat when ending your fast, and the best foods to consume during your regular eating windows.

Foods You Can Eat While Fasting

While fasting implies abstinence from food, there are certain things that you can still devour without putting a dent in your regimen.

Here are some of those more forgiving foods:

- **Plain old water:** You can consume plain water to keep yourself hydrated during a fast without adding to the calorie count.

- **Tea and coffee:** Tea and coffee (without added sugar, milk, or cream) can be consumed during a fast. Black coffee might actually enhance the benefits of IF since it is demonstrated to support healthy blood sugar levels over the long term.

- **Apple cider vinegar (diluted):** Apple cider vinegar can be consumed during fasting and eating windows. Along with its antimicrobial and antioxidant properties, ACV can enhance the benefits of IF by supporting healthy blood sugar and digestion and keeping a person hydrated during a fast.

- **Bone broth:** A bone (or veggie) broth is highly recommended during IF as it supplies the body with essential amino acids as well as other minerals and vitamins while instilling a feeling of being full. However, be highly aware of canned or store-bought broth varieties containing artificial flavors and preservatives. Instead, stir up a nice homemade broth with a little bit of sea salt to promote water retention during fasting.

Foods to Eat When Ending a Fast

While you may think that the world is yours once your fasting period ends, remember that it is always a good practice to be mindful of what you are putting in your body to build on the benefits of fasting you just banked on.

The last thing you want to do is spoil everything you've just earned through fasting by gobbling a huge pizza or feeding on an extra-large burger with fries.

Sounds tempting… but it isn't recommended.

What's more, fasting intermittently means that you have a relatively narrower eating window than normal. If you don't eat well during these windows of opportunity, you might put yourself at the risk of facing malnutrition, which can lead to a host of undesirable health conditions.

Eating after you've fasted for a considerable amount of time can be challenging in a few ways. Not only do you have to ensure that you're eating nutrient-dense food, but you must also be cautious of putting too much too soon on your digestive system. It takes about 20 minutes to feel satisfied after eating a meal, so it is easy to overeat, especially after a longer fasting period. Because of that, it is suggested to break your fast with a smaller meal or snack about 30 minutes before having your normal size lunch or dinner. In this way, you will help your organs and their digestive functions too.

This is why I include a list of foods that you can refer to when the time comes to finally eat something:

- **Nuts and Seeds:** Almonds, walnuts, flax seeds, chia seeds are great sources of healthy fats. Perhaps a quick and easy way to restore your energy levels without spiking the glucose levels in the blood is to consume a handful of nuts.

- **Veggies and Salads:** Most of us don't need another long and boring lesson on the importance of consuming vegetables, but here it is again. (I promise to keep it short, though!) While all veggies are good for health, some starchy ones, such as sweet potatoes, can be a great source of resistant starches when breaking a fast. Just make sure that you cook them up thoroughly.

- **Soups:** Soups and broths aren't only good when you're fasting but can also be a great source of nutrients and vitamins when you're finally ready to eat again. While a simple veggie or bone broth can be your best friend during fasting, you can add a bunch of stuff like lentils, tofu or pasta to spice it up for the post-fasting period.

- **Smoothies:** These are a great way to give your body the nutrient punch it needs after fasting for several hours. What's more, smoothies are always fun to make since you can throw together almost anything and stir up a nutritious yet delicious drink within minutes. Not a vegetable person? Add in some romaine lettuce or spinach in your blend to prevent missing out on the benefits of these leafy greens without having to consume a bowl full of baked veggies instead.

70

- **Fermented Foods:** foods such as unsweetened yogurt and kefir are a great source of probiotics that your gut will thank you over a million times for. Yogurt also contains almost all the nutrients that our bodies need, including but not limited to calcium, B vitamins, proteins, phosphorus, and vitamin D. It is a precious source of trace minerals. It is found to be particularly beneficial for osteoporosis and digestive health.

- **Fruits (Fresh & Dried):** To keep it light on your gut, you can also break your fast with fruits such as watermelon, grapes, and honeydew. These are ideal because they contain a high water content to combat dehydration and are easily digestible. If you want some inspiration from folks in other parts of the world, don't look beyond the Middle East and Arabia. People inhabiting these regions prefer to break their fasts with dates which are a dense source of nutrients, and restore energy levels after a long fast. If dates are not your thing, try dried apricots or raisins for similar effects.

- **Healthy Fats:** Breaking your fast with healthy fats such as eggs, avocados, coconut and olive oil, ghee, and grass-fed butter will ensure that your digestive system is not overwhelmed and that you get the right nutrients that your body craves for after a fast. Egg is among the finest sources of fats: boiled, pouched, and deviled eggs are a perfect way to add proteins and essential micronutrients to the diet.

Super Foods to Eat During the Eating Window

Mediterranean-style diets are considered the healthiest option. They are based primarily on lots of vegetables and fruits, whole grains, nuts and seeds, fish and lean poultry, olive oil, and yes, red wine seems to be a common inclusion. What's missing: meats loaded with saturated fats and processed foods high in sugar, salt, or both. Fried foods are minimal.

A Mediterranean diet pyramid was developed by the Harvard School of Public Health, in collaboration with the World Health Organization (WHO), and Boston-based Oldways, a nonprofit food, and nutrition advisory service:

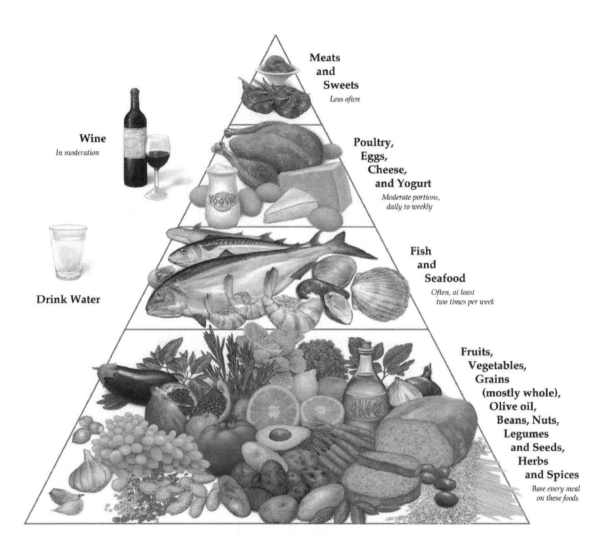

However, consistency is the key, and if 80% of your food choices come from nutritious and balanced foods, that would be great. That will add even more benefits on top of IF and help you reach your goals faster. So, let's find out which foods you should make the mainstays of your regular diet.

Whole Grains

Choosing whole grains is part of a clean and healthy diet. Their easy digestion and cleansing properties make them ideal for the intermittent fast. They are high in protein and fiber. Instead of the conventional wheat and oats, try bulgar, amaranth, and flax.

Legumes and Beans

Adapting the IF lifestyle might prompt you to fall in love with legumes and beans rich in low-calorie carbs that can supply you with enough energy for your daily activities. This makes them vital additions to your eating plan. Also, foods that belong to the legume and bean family, including black beans, lentils, peas, and chickpeas, can significantly reduce your body weight even if you do not restrict your calorie intake.

Eggs

We all know how high in protein eggs are, but one of the key benefits of eggs in an intermittent fasting eating pattern is how versatile they are. They are a quick snack that can be prepared in minutes. You are also not limited to hard boiled eggs. They may be blended and prepared in a variety of ways, guaranteeing that you never eat the same meal twice.

Fish

Fish is a weight-loss miracle food. Six to eight ounces of fish per week is recommended per dietary guidelines. Fish is nutrient-dense and a good source of fats and proteins. You won't need supplements if you eat fish frequently, as it's rich in vitamin D and omega-3 fatty acids (DHA) that are dairy-free. You'll be more attentive and able to think clearly as a result. You'll be more productive and less stressed.

Leafy Greens

Leafy green veggies are the type of food we remember our parents telling us to eat. As we all know, leafy greens are filled with beneficial elements. Kale, broccoli, lettuce, etc., are high in fiber. As you may know, fiber keeps your digestive system moving when you are constipated. You will experience it if you undertake an intermittent fast. It is even more vital to eat these vegetables to maintain your gut health in this circumstance. Fiber also helps you feel fuller between meals.

Sweet Potato

Sweet potato is one of the best options for those who want to do intermittent fasting. It serves as a source of healthy fiber and carbohydrates, generating a feeling of satiety. They're also high in carotenoids, a type of antioxidant that may lower your risk of certain cancers. Sweet potatoes do not raise blood sugar levels despite their sweet flavor. Surprisingly, they may help blood sugar control in people with type 2 diabetes. Choose the baked or roasted version.

Avocado

You may be wondering why avocado is on this list when it is so high in fat. But you must realize that fasting can be taxing on your body, so you must eat meals that will keep you going. Avocado is high in monounsaturated fat, which helps those who become hungry easily. It keeps you full longer. You won't reach for a snack. Avocado is a great addition to any breakfast or lunch meal. Those who eat it during breakfast can go longer periods without feeling hungry.

Assorted Berries

Nothing beats eating fresh berries first thing in the morning. They're high in antioxidants and essential elements that keep your body healthy. Strawberries, raspberries, blueberries, and gooseberries are all excellent sources of antioxidants. To prepare a smoothie, simply combine them with some milk or yogurt in a blender. According to research, those who ate berries on a regular basis were able to maintain their ideal body weight and did not gain excessive weight over time.

Foods to Avoid for Best Results

The intermittent fasting approach calls for you to avoid, or at least significantly reduce, the following foods:

- **White starchy foods.** This includes pasta and potatoes. Starch is metabolized as glucose and immediately goes into fat stores.

- **Foods loaded with carbs.** White bread, or anything baked, is usually loaded with many carbs.

- **Greasy foods.** Deep-fried and very greasy foods, while tasty, are high in unhealthy fats. These types of fats lead to high cholesterol. These foods are the number one enemy for blood vessel health. They generally lead to poor circulation.

- **Salty foods.** There's nothing wrong with salt unless you eat too much of it. Salting foods to taste is fine. However, excessively salty foods are not only addictive, but they affect your blood pressure and heart health. It's best to switch to sea salt as it contains less sodium.

- **Sugary drinks and alcohol.** By "sugary," we mean things like sodas and iced teas. These are loaded with sugar and other chemicals. Also, alcoholic beverages end up accumulating fat in a heartbeat. Consuming moderate amounts of alcohol is perfectly fine (1–2 drinks per week). In fact, a glass of wine will do a great number to your heart. However, it's excessive alcohol consumption that leads to increased fat gains. This is because alcohol is metabolized by the body the same way sugar is. So, this implies you'll be packing on extra glucose in your system.

Supplements and Intermittent Fasting

Even when a person is on a normal diet, they are always at a risk of nutritional deficiency. Essential micronutrients like vitamins and minerals are important for all the metabolic processes occurring in the body. Due to a poor and unhealthy diet, we fail to consume enough of these nutrients and gradually suffer health problems due to these deficiencies. It is not the amount of food that matters nor the caloric content. It is the type of food that ensures a balanced intake of vitamin A, B, C, D, E, and K. Some minerals like sodium, calcium, potassium, magnesium, and phosphorus are also required for the body to carry out both catabolic and anabolic activities. But the diets we consume usually do not include these elements in sufficient amounts, or we fail to add vitamin or mineral-rich food to our diet.

Women who cross the age of 50 are going through various bodily changes, and they are the ones who need these elements the most. As the body and mind both lose their capacity to regulate an enhanced absorption of that micronutrient, it is important to consume them in large amounts to increase their bioavailability. To provide maximum micronutrients to elderly women, experts recommend consuming different types of supplements to regulate metabolism. These supplements are considered best to consume on the intermittent fasting program, as they prevent multiple possible nutritional deficiencies in women over 50.

Multivitamins

Vitamins are divided into two main categories: water-soluble and fat-soluble vitamins. Water-soluble vitamins like Vitamin C are quickly digested and used in the body. Therefore, they should be consumed on a regular daily basis. However, the fat-soluble vitamins are more long-lasting. Since a woman's body requires different types of vitamins, it is suggested to take multivitamin supplements.

Fish Oil

Fish and algae oil tablets and ampules are readily available on the market, and they can be consumed orally. These oils are essentially low on calories, but they contain omega-3 and omega-6 fatty acids. These are effective in lowering blood cholesterol levels and preventing heart diseases, which are common among people over the age of 50. Omegas are largely present in seafood, but not everyone consumes enough seafood to meet their needs, so omega supplements provide a better alternative to food-sourced omegas.

Other Micronutrients

Every micronutrient plays a different function in the body. Depending on one's diet, lifestyle, and genetic makeup, people may suffer from deficiency of a particular micronutrient. For example, vitamin D deficiency is quite common in women, which can result in irritability, insomnia, and bone weakness. Similarly, deficiency of calcium also leads to bone weakness. So, a person can go for specific micronutrients that are largely available in different supplements. Tablets of vitamin C, vitamin B complex, and others are available in supplement form.

Pure Collagen

After the age of 50, women usually suffer from excess hair loss, wrinkling, and dryness of the skin. Good use of collagen supplements is important to keep the hair and skin as young as ever. When consumed in a small amount regularly, these supplements can give your skin a new life and your hair good growth.

Probiotics and prebiotics

The human gut system works mainly due to the presence of thousands of micro-bacteria that create a friendly microbiome within the digestive tract. When a person suffers from nutritional deficiencies and weakness, this microbiome also suffers. Prolonged fasting and eating unhealthy food are also responsible for destroying gut bacteria. Therefore, the intake of probiotics and prebiotics is absolutely necessary. Both supplements strengthen the gut biome and help achieve better digestion, assimilation, and absorption of the consumed food. Together, prebiotic fibers and probiotic bacteria can help keep the digestive system healthy and working. Both are available in pills and other supplements. Use these supplements according to the dose suggested by your health expert.

Creatine

Creatine is an important element that supports the building and repair of muscles. The supplement is more useful for people who want to keep their muscles in shape. Women who work out or are into sports can consume creatine as a supplement in some amount to keep the muscles strong and healthy. Creatine can be useful if you need more energy for your workouts.

Chapter Summary

- There are two considerations for proper food choices: what to eat and when to eat.

- In considering the first question, there are simple guidelines to follow: reduce intake of refined grains and sugars, moderate protein consumption, increase natural fats and fiber, choose natural, unprocessed foods.

- In considering the second question, balance insulin-dominant periods with insulin-deficient periods. Balance your feeding and fasting. Eating continuously is a recipe for weight gain. IF is a very effective way to deal with when to eat.

- You can break the fast by eating a small portion of nuts or salad before having a bigger meal.

- Supplements may help fasters fill nutrient shortages associated with fasting.

When you stop eating for an extended time, you will experience various adverse effects. These can be excruciating at first, but if you learn how to really deal with them, you will be able to persist with IF and reap the rewards. I will provide more suggestions in the next chapter.

CHAPTER 6: HOW TO DEAL WITH CHALLENGES AND SIDE EFFECTS

Think about it this way: people don't go from couch potato to triathlete overnight. Your body needs time to acclimate to any extreme changes. So you're going to experience some side effects when you suddenly stop eating for long periods of time.

–Stephanie Ferrari, a registered dietitian

There are pros and cons of everything, and intermittent fasting is no exception. It is a complete lifestyle change, and hence making the transition can be difficult for some people. This chapter will help you understand the problems you can face and how to deal with them.

While following intermittent fasting, you can face mild symptoms like headache, cravings, hunger pangs, bloating, constipation, etc. If you encounter such issues, there is no reason to worry as these aren't big or permanent problems. These issues occur because you are making a change in your lifestyle. There are ways to deal with these challenges and set yourself up for success.

Managing Hunger

The most difficult challenge is the hunger problem. Let's face it: we are human beings, and our bodies need food to survive. From the time we were babies, we have been taught to eat when hunger strikes. For 50 years or more, your body has followed this pattern. You can't expect to unlearn it in a day. As we have taught our body to grab a bite when we are famished, similarly, we have to train our body to manage hunger by breaking this pattern. You have to go very slowly. Experts say that you must follow the same routine for at least 21 days to form a habit. I'm sure you have all heard that. Rather than the number of days, though, you should just focus on consistency.

Another concept that I have learned to value over time is integrity and grit. In fact, you can find 'grit' in integrity, both literally and figuratively. Integrity is the quality of being serious and steady with respect to your actions and principles. It means sticking to principles and ideas and following them. It does require grit. And when grit is pursued over time with dedication and genuineness, it simply becomes integrity. So yes, at times, all you need is that. That means if you really want something, learning a new pattern is fairly easy. Let's discuss some simple ways in which you could suppress your appetite.

Water, Water, and More Water

This is the most effortless hack for taking care of hunger pangs. It is a natural hunger suppressant. You don't even have to worry about calories since water has none. Hunger is basically a signal sent by our stomach to the brain that it's empty. So, when you fill your stomach with water, you are conning your tummy into believing that it is full. Your brain gets a message from your stomach, "Hey, I am full now. We can stop bothering this person." You see, it's the most effective and easiest method to overcome this challenge. Also, sometimes we may feel hungry when what our body actually needs is water.

If you don't like to drink plain water, squeeze a lemon into it. Lemon water is a great detox. As they say, "When life throws lemons at you, make lemonade!"

Apple Cider Vinegar Drink

This magical potion is an elixir. I mentioned this in a previous chapter, but here I will go into a little more detail to help you internalize the essential goodness of apple cider vinegar. It has minimal calories, so you are safe from a calorie perspective. Apple cider vinegar is nothing but a fermented juice obtained from crushing apples. You might be happy to know that apple cider vinegar has many health benefits like promoting satiety, weight loss, controlling blood sugar and blood pressure, increasing metabolism, promoting digestion, etc. That's a big list, isn't it?

You should always consume apple cider vinegar in a diluted form. Add one teaspoon to a glass of water and gulp it like some critical medicine. You can drink it on an empty stomach in the morning or at night before bedtime. When you drink it in the morning, you will have fewer cravings throughout the day, and you can easily survive the fasting period. One study found out that apple cider vinegar, when taken at night before bedtime, significantly stabilizes fasting blood sugar in the morning.

When you buy apple cider vinegar, remember to look for only the organic, raw, and unfiltered kind with a label that says, "with the 'mother.'" This is the purest form of apple cider vinegar and provides maximum health benefits. Also, brush your teeth or rinse your mouth after a drink because acetic acid may cause dental problems if you don't.

Black Coffee, Black Tea, or Organic Teas

Coffee and tea are stimulants that work as appetite suppressants. A hormone named cholecystokinin (CCK) is released after eating, slowing stomach emptying and promoting satiety. Black coffee stimulates the release of CCK. Coffee and tea also promote fat burning, so when fat stores are burned, you get a supply of energy during your fasting period.

You may also try organic teas like green tea, which has an antioxidant named Epigallocatechin gallate (EGCG), which increases metabolism by burning glycogen and fats stores for energy.

Just be mindful of not over-drinking stimulants as they also aggravate anxiety. Postmenopausal women already know how anxiety can be a hair ripping experience. To keep anxiety levels low, drink only one cup of black coffee, black tea, or organic tea. That will do the trick of decreasing appetite. But of course, if you can handle your caffeine, go ahead and pour yourself another. These drinks have many antioxidants that are naturally anti-aging and significantly bring down daily inflammation levels.

Cumin Seed Water

This is another excellent, low-calorie remedy for hunger. Cumin water is a war hero when it comes to controlling hunger issues and cravings. It will keep you off processed foods for a longer time. This potion also accelerates the fat-burning process.

Simply soak a teaspoon of cumin seeds in a glass of water overnight and drink it the next morning. Other than controlling your hunger, they work by stabilizing a lot of things in your body, from your insulin to your inflammation. So, adding them to your morning schedule can be very helpful for feeling great throughout the day.

Fenugreek Seeds

Fenugreek seeds are extremely filling due to their fiber content. Even a teaspoon of soaked fenugreek seeds in the morning shall keep you satiated for a longer time. Soak a teaspoon of these seeds overnight. Eat them first thing in the morning, along with the water they were soaked in. Another wonderful thing about soaked fenugreek seeds is that they will improve your metabolic health in general. They are often recommended to diabetics, too.

These little seeds can be super effective when it comes to digestion. In fact, those who deal with acidity as a chronic condition might find them even more helpful. They will ease you into a good night at the end of the day. However, it's a little difficult to find the seeds in supermarket stores. Fenugreek seeds can be added to tea or heated water. Fenugreek provides fiber and may help suppress hunger, which is important during a fast. Note that 1 tsp of fenugreek contains around 12 calories, so you may want to use less.

Divert Your Mind

Sometimes stress can also trigger hunger, especially if you are an emotional eater. Or you could even be a creature of habit. If you are habituated to eating breakfast, you will feel hungry even if you actually aren't. And most certainly, you will know the difference between a pang of real hunger and a perceived one. You only need to pay close attention to your body. If this is the case, you can practice diverting your mind from food. Go for a walk, read a book, or write in your journal. Do any enjoyable activity that will shift your focus from eating.

Keep all the tempting foods out of sight. Don't open the fridge every now and then. If possible, minimize your trips to the kitchen. If you are cooking meals for your feeding period, read and reread your goal to yourself while cooking. Do some household activities such as cleaning, organizing your wardrobe, or even gardening. If you are a working woman, immerse yourself in your work tasks. When your mind is busy, you will not think about food. Request your colleagues not to offer you any snacks during the fasting period.

Practice meditation. Sit still and observe your breath. Try to bring your attention to the present moment. Make a mental shift, and just take it easy!

And think about hunger like waves: they will come, and they will soon disappear.

Headache

It is also a common problem that people face. There is nothing to worry about the headaches as they occur when going through sugar withdrawal systems.

Our lifestyle has become such that our dependency on a carbohydrate-rich diet has increased significantly. We also keep consuming meals at frequent intervals, and hence our body keeps getting glucose supply at short intervals. Our body loves glucose fuel as it is easy to burn and can be absorbed by the cells directly. However, being easy doesn't make it good. It leaves a lot of waste and residue in the body.

When you begin intermittent fasting, you block the regular supply of glucose fuel. Your body requires energy dump at short intervals. It can also derive energy from the fat stores, but it is difficult to burn fuel, and hence your brain starts giving you signals to eat frequently in the form of a headache. If you don't start eating frequently, your body would have no other option than to switch to fat fuel in the body. It is a clean fuel that leaves no toxic waste and residue. It would make you slimmer and also help in getting rid of diseases.

The easy way to counter the headaches is to have unsweetened black tea or coffee. These beverages help deal with headaches and don't add any calories to your system. You can have them without breaking your fast. However, don't become overly dependent on coffee and tea. Taking too much caffeine can destabilize the quality of your sleep, resulting in stress and anxiety that may well promote rebound weight gain.

Cravings

Cravings can mean a lot of different things for men, but they have a unique meaning when it comes to women. Food cravings can arise in women due to emotional needs or psychological distress. Women can find great solace in food, especially in sweets and desserts.

However, in general, craving is bad, and the biggest cause of food craving is the intake of sweets. Candies, chocolates, cookies, carbonated beverages, and other such things that are high in sugar content can cause sugar cravings. One must always try to stay away from such things.

The best way to deal with this problem is to completely abstain from high sugar foods. If possible, staying away from high-carb food items is highly advisable as they also have a lot of sugar. You must try to avoid processed food items as much as possible.

Eat food items that are high in healthy fats and proteins. The higher the fat and protein content in your food, the lower will be your food cravings and these nutrients take a lot of time to get processed in the gut. Your gut remains pleasantly engaged and can clean itself properly.

Irritability

It's common to feel a little cranky because of a drop in your blood sugar levels. This can get worse when coupled with other side effects like low energy and cravings. The best way to deal with this is by avoiding people or situations that will make you feel more annoyed and instead focusing on the things that will make you happy.

Frequent Trips to the Toilet

It is not very unusual for people to feel the frequent need to urinate when they begin their fasting routine. However, there is no need to worry as it is common for most weight loss programs. When you start any weight loss program and reduce your calorie intake, your body starts the protective mechanism.

It tries to lower energy needs. The water in your body, apart from keeping you hydrated, also helps regulate body temperature. However, as soon as you lower your calorie intake, the body starts dumping the water to compensate for the energy deficit. But there is nothing to worry about as this is a temporary phenomenon, and the water levels in your body will be back soon.

When you begin fasting, your body also starts cleaning itself of the toxins, and that also causes frequent urination. As long as you do not feel any discomfort or the trips haven't increased a lot, it should not worry you much.

You should keep drinking lots of water to compensate for the loss. If hypertension or other medical issues are not there, you should even try water with a pinch of sea salt. It helps replenish the loss of minerals that occurs due to excessive urination.

Heartburn, Bloating, and Constipation

Heartburn and bloating are common issues you may face when you begin fasting. The reasons for bloating are simple: your gut keeps releasing the digestive juices at regular intervals but doesn't get anything to digest that causes the problem. However, this is a very temporary phenomenon as your gut would easily adjust to your new eating schedules, and the problem would subside.

Heartburn is also part of the same process, but it causes the most discomfort. The good thing is that it wouldn't last long. As soon as the release of digestive juices gets timed, bloating and heartburn will subside.

Constipation, on the other hand, can be a problem for many. The main reason for constipation isn't fasting but intake of improper food. It is a fact that your food intake may reduce when you begin intermittent fasting as your number of meals goes down. However, if you don't include high-fiber food items in your meals, your gut wouldn't have much to process. This can cause constipation that may trouble you a lot.

The best way to avoid it is to have fiber-rich food. Increase the salads and fiber-rich food in your meals, and you would face no such issue. The important thing to remember is that you need to understand the problems you face and try to find the solution. Don't stick to a particular thing but try to find your best routine.

Intermittent fasting may become a big change in your life. You will have to make a few adjustments to welcome this change. It will be easy for you and even beneficial if you start adjusting to accommodate them. Don't be stubborn or a stickler for rules. Try to find your rhythm and flow with it.

Feeling Cold

When you fast, your blood flow to your fat store increases, resulting in cold toes and fingers; this is known as adipose tissue blood flow, and it's essential for moving fat to your muscles, where it's burned for energy. A decline in your blood sugar levels may also be responsible for the increased sensitivity to cold. You can combat this feeling of coldness with hot showers, sipping hot tea, or dressing up in layered clothing. Where possible, stay indoors for longer.

Chapter Summary

- It's a good idea to be aware of the possible side effects you may encounter as you fast.

- While you may be very hungry at first, just keep busy, stay hydrated, and stay strong. As your body adjusts to fasting, the hunger usually subsides.

- Fasting can boost your energy, focus, and productivity. Your body may take some time to acclimate to your new fasting schedule. As a result, some people encounter fatigue and headache at the beginning. Keep going; these side effects usually subside within a week or two.

- Some people may suffer from constipation or go to the bathroom less frequently than usual. You might be eating less naturally because your feeding window is shorter. When you fast longer, you consume less food, so you go less frequently. What you eat and how much water you drink could also influence how regularly you go. When you are eating for a short period, prioritize foods high in fiber, vitamins, protein, and water.

- It is not surprising if you get to a point where you are overly dependent on coffee and tea. Taking too much caffeine can destabilize the quality of your sleep, resulting in stress and anxiety that may well promote rebound weight gain.

- If you do experience one of these side effects, just know that they will go away! Just like dieting, you'll experience hunger, cravings, irritability, bowel movements, and many other side effects when you first start. After a while, your body will adjust, and you'll feel fantastic.

We, as humans, are bound to make mistakes. The same goes for an IF regimen whose flexibility makes it more prone to people making some serious blunders all the time. What are these, and how to avoid them? Let's find out in the next chapter.

CHAPTER 7: COMMON MISTAKES TO AVOID

Success lies in one's ability to learn from mistakes.

–Dr Prem Jagyasi

When you are looking to make any significant adjustments in your life, it can take time to discover exactly how to do it in the best ways possible. Many people will make mistakes and have some setbacks as they seek to improve their health through intermittent fasting. Some of these mistakes are minor and can easily be overcome, whereas others may be dangerous and could cause severe repercussions if they are not caught in time.

In this chapter, we will explore common mistakes that people tend to make when they are on the intermittent fasting eating plan. We will also explore why these mistakes are made and how they can be avoided. It is important that you read through this chapter before you actually commit to the eating pattern itself. That way, you can ensure that you are avoiding any potential mistakes beforehand. This will help you avoid unwanted problems and achieve your results with greater success and fewer setbacks.

Switching Too Fast

A significant number of people fail to comply with their new eating patterns because they attempt to go too hard too fast. Trying to jump too quickly can result in feeling too extreme of a departure from your normal. As a result, both psychologically and physically, you are put under a significant amount of stress from your new eating pattern. This can lead to you feeling like the eating pattern is not actually effective and like you are suffering more than you are benefitting from it.

If you eat regularly and snack frequently, switching to the intermittent fasting eating pattern will take time and patience. I cannot stress the importance of your transition period enough.

It is not uncommon to want to jump off the deep end when making a lifestyle change. We often want to experience great results right away and are excited about the switch. However, after a few days, it can feel stressful. Because you didn't give your mind and body enough time to adapt to the changes, you ditch your new diet in favor of more comfortable things.

Fasting should always be acclimated to over a period of time. There is no set period; it needs to be done based on what feels right for you and your body. If you are not properly listening to your body and its needs, you will end up suffering in major ways. Especially with an eating pattern like intermittent fasting, letting yourself adapt to the changes and listening to your body's needs can ensure that you are not neglecting your body in favor of strictly following someone else's guide on what to do.

Simply start by lowering the number of snacks you have in a day. The snacks have not only become a need of the body, but they are also a part of the habit. In a day, there are numerous instances when we eat tit-bits that we don't care about. We sip cold drinks and sweetened beverages and eat chips, cookies, bagels, donuts, burgers, pizzas simply because they are in front of us or accessible. We have made food an excuse to take breaks. This habit will have to be broken if you want to move on the path of good health.

Choosing the Wrong Plan for Your Lifestyle

It is not uncommon to forget the importance of picking a fasting cycle that actually fits with your lifestyle and then fitting it in. Trying to fast to a cycle that does not fit with your lifestyle will ultimately result in you feeling inconvenienced by your eating pattern and struggling to maintain it.

Often, the way we naturally eat is in accordance with what we feel fits into our lifestyle in the best way possible. So, if you look at your present diet and notice that there are a lot of convenience meals and they happen all throughout the day, you can conclude two things: you are busy, and you eat when you can. Picking a diet that allows you to eat when you can is important in helping you stick to it. It is also important that you begin searching for healthier convenience options to get the most out of your eating pattern.

Anytime you make a lifestyle change, such as with your diet, you need to consider your lifestyle. In an ideal world, you may be able to adapt everything to suit your dreamy needs completely. However, there are likely many aspects of your lifestyle in the real world that are simply not practical to adjust. Picking an eating pattern that suits your lifestyle rather than picking a lifestyle that suits your eating pattern makes far more sense.

Taking the time to actually document what your present eating habits are like before you embark on your intermittent fasting diet is a great way to begin. Focus on what you are already eating and how often and consider eating patterns that will serve your lifestyle. You should also consider your activity levels and how much food you truly need at certain times of the day. For example, if you have a spin class every morning, fasting until noon might not be a good idea as you could end up hungry and exhausted after your class. Choosing the eating pattern that fits your lifestyle will help you maintain your eating pattern so you can continue receiving great results from it.

Eating Too Much or Not Enough

Focusing on what you are eating and how much you are eating is important. This is one of the biggest reasons why a gradual and intentional transition can be helpful. If you are used to eating throughout the entire day, eating the same amount in a shorter window can be challenging. You may find yourself feeling stuffed and far too full to actually sustain that amount of eating on a day-to-day basis. As a result, you may find yourself not eating enough.

91

If you are new to intermittent fasting and you take the leap too quickly, it is not unusual to find yourself scarfing down as much food as you possibly can the moment your eating window opens back up. As a result, you find yourself feeling sick, too full, and uncomfortable. Your body also struggles to process and digest that much food after fasting for any given period of time. This can be even harder on your body if you have been using a more intense fast and then you stuff yourself. If you find yourself doing this, it may be a sign that you have transitioned too quickly and that you need to slow down and back off.

You might also find yourself not eating enough. Attempting to eat the same amount that you typically eat in 12-16 hours in just 8-12 hours can be challenging. It may not sound so drastic on paper, but if you are not hungry, you may simply not feel like eating. As a result, you may feel compelled to skip meals. This can lead to you not getting enough calories and nutrition daily. In the end, you find yourself not eating enough and feeling unsatisfied during your fasting windows.

The best way to combat this is to begin practicing making healthier calorie-dense foods before you actually start intermittent fasting. Learning what recipes you can make and how much each meal needs to have to help you reach your goals is a great way to get yourself ready and show yourself what it truly takes to succeed. Then, begin gradually shortening your eating window and giving yourself the time to work up to eating enough during those eating windows without overeating. In the end, you will find yourself feeling amazing and not feeling unsatisfied or overeating as you maintain your eating pattern.

Your Food Choices Are Not Healthy Enough

Even if you are eating according to the keto diet or any other dietary style while intermittent fasting, it is not uncommon to find yourself eating the wrong food choices. Simply knowing what to eat and what to avoid is not enough. You need to spend some time getting to understand what specific vitamins and minerals you need to thrive. That way, you can eat a diet rich in these specific nutrients. Then, you can trust that your body has everything that it needs to thrive on your diet.

Even though intermittent fasting does not technically outline what you should and should not eat, it is not a one-size-fits-all eating pattern that can help you lose weight while eating anything you want. In other words, excessive amounts of junk foods will still harm you, even if you're eating during the right windows.

You must choose a diet that will help you maintain everything you need to function optimally. You can even combine intermittent fasting with another diet such as the keto diet, the Mediterranean diet, or any other diet that supports you in eating healthfully. Following the guidelines of these healthier diets ensures that you are incorporating the proper nutrients into your diet to stay healthy.

Eating the right nutrients is essential as it will support your body in healthy hormonal balance and bodily functions. This is how you can keep your organs functioning effectively so that everything works the way it should. As a result, you end up feeling healthier and experiencing greater benefits from your diet. You must focus on this if you want to succeed with your intermittent fasting eating pattern.

Not Drinking Enough Fluids

Many people do not realize how much hydration their foods actually give them on a day-to-day basis. Foods like fruits and vegetables are filled with hydration that supports your body in healthy functions. If you are not eating as much, you can guarantee that you are not getting as much hydration as you need to. This means that you need to focus on increasing your hydration levels.

When dehydrated, you can experience many unwanted symptoms that can make intermittent fasting a challenge. Increased headaches, muscle cramping, and increased hunger are all side effects of dehydration. A great way to combat dehydration is to make sure that you keep water nearby and sip it often. At least once every half an hour you should have a good drink of water. This will ensure that you get plenty of fresh water into your system.

Other ways to maintain your hydration levels include drinking low-calorie sports drinks, bone broth, and tea. Essentially, drinking low-calorie drinks throughout the day can be extremely helpful in supporting your health. Make sure that you do not exceed your fasting calorie maximum, however, or you will stop gaining the benefits of fasting. Water should always be your first choice above any other drinks to maintain your hydration. However, including some of the others from time to time can support you and keep things interesting so that you can stay hydrated but not bored.

If you begin to experience any symptoms of dehydration, make sure that you immediately begin increasing the amount of water that you are drinking. Dehydration can lead to far more serious side effects beyond headaches and muscle cramps if you are not careful. If you find that you are prone to not drinking enough water daily, consider setting a reminder on your phone that keeps you drinking plenty throughout the day.

The best way to tell that you are staying hydrated is to pay attention to how frequently you are peeing. If you are staying in a healthy range of hydration, you should be peeing at least once every single hour. If you aren't, this means that you need to be drinking more water, even if you aren't experiencing any side effects of dehydration. Typically, if you have already begun experiencing side effects, you have waited too long. You want to maintain healthy hydration without waiting for symptoms like headaches and muscle aches to inform you that it is time to start drinking more. This ensures that your body stays happy and healthy and that you are not causing unnecessary suffering or stress to your body throughout the day.

Giving Up Too Quickly

Many people assume that eating on the intermittent fasting eating pattern means seeing the benefits of their eating habits immediately. This is not the case. While intermittent fasting typically offers great results fairly quickly, it takes some time for these results to begin appearing. The exact amount of time depends on many factors. How long it has taken you to transition, what and how you are eating during eating windows, and how much activity you are getting throughout the day all contribute to your results.

You might feel compelled to quickly give up if you do not begin noticing your desired results right away, but trust that this will not help you. Some people require several weeks before they really begin seeing the benefits of their dieting. This does not mean that it is not working; it simply means that it has taken them some time to find the right balance to gain their desired results and stay healthy.

If you feel like throwing in the towel, first take a few minutes to consider what you are doing and how it may negatively impact your results. A great way to do this is to try using your food diary again. For a few days, track how you are eating in accordance with the intermittent fasting diet and what it is doing for you. Get a clear idea of how much you are eating, what you are eating, and when you are eating it. Also, track the amount of physical activity that you are doing on a daily basis.

By tracking your food intake and exercise levels, you might find that you are not experiencing the results you desire because you are eating too much or not enough compared to the amount of energy you are spending each day. Then, you can easily work towards adjusting your diet to find a balance that supports you in getting everything you need and seeing the results you desire.

In most cases, intermittent fasting eating patterns are not working because they are not being used correctly for an individual person. Although the general requirements are somewhat the same, each of us has unique needs based on our lifestyles and our unique makeup. If you are willing to invest time in finding the right balance for yourself, you can guarantee that you can overcome this and experience great results from your fasting.

Getting Too Intense or Pushing It

If you are really focused on achieving your desired results, you might feel compelled to push your eating pattern further than what is reasonable for you—for example, attempting to take on too intense of a fasting cycle or trying to do more than your body can reasonably handle. It is not uncommon for people to try and push themselves beyond reasonable measures to achieve their desired results. Unfortunately, this rarely results in them achieving what they actually set out to achieve. It can also have severe consequences.

At the end of the day, listening to your body and paying attention to exactly what it needs is important. You need to be taking care of yourself through proper nutrition and proper exercise levels. You also need to balance these two to serve your body, rather than in a way that leads to you feeling sick and unwell. If you push your body too far, the negative consequences can be severe and long-lasting. In some cases, they may even be life-threatening.

In some cases, pushing your body to a certain extent is necessary. For example, if you are seeking to tone your body, you want to push yourself to work out enough that your workouts are effective. However, if you are pushing yourself to the point that you are beginning to experience negative side effects from your diet, you need to scale back. While certain side effects are fairly normal early on, experiencing intense side effects, having side effects that don't go away, or having them return is not good. You want to maintain and minimize your side effects, not constantly living alongside them. After all, what is the point of adjusting your eating pattern and lifestyle to serve your health if you are not actually feeling healthy while you do it?

Make sure that you check in with yourself daily to see to it that your physical needs are being met. That way, if anything begins to feel excessive or any symptoms begin to increase, you can focus on minimizing or eliminating them right away. Paying close attention to your needs and

96

looking at your goals long-term rather than trying to reach them immediately is the best way to ensure that you reach your health goals without actually compromising your health while attempting to do so. In the end, you will feel much better about doing it this way.

Not Exercising When Intermittent Fasting

Try fitting some form of physical activity into your busy schedule, even if it's just taking a brisk walk around the neighborhood after dinner! And remember, sleeping for less than seven hours per night has been linked with obesity and other chronic diseases, so try to get those eight recommended hours each day! More advice on exercise will be provided in Chapter 9.

***

Chapter Summary

- While there is extensive guidance available on how to approach IF, we can all make mistakes sometimes. This is especially relevant since IF allows a significant amount of wiggle room for experimentation, implying that people may be making some mistakes with regard to the practice, although unintentionally.

- There is no one-size-fits-all intermittent fasting plan. What might work for someone else may not work for you. You need to find the IF routine that best suits your body and lifestyle.

- Your body needs time to adjust to fasting intermittently, don't push it too hard, or you'll cause it to work on the side of giving up!

- Do not put yourself into unnecessary trouble by choosing an IF regimen that contradicts how you normally go about your day. Because if you do so, you're setting yourself up for some real headache.

- Dehydration can cause lethargy, muscle weakness, headaches, and dizziness. And these can highly affect a person when they're already fasting. You can drink water during and after the fasting period or enjoy a cup of black tea or coffee, depending on your mood.

- If you cannot control yourself while fasting, then it might be best for you to take small portions of food during each fast period instead of devouring everything in sight during one big feast. This will help reduce the number of calories consumed and slow down weight gain or loss if this is happening quickly due to intermittent fasting.

- It's crucial to continue being physically active even while intermittent fasting. Exercise helps burn calories and promote better health, which is beneficial when losing weight or maintaining a healthy lifestyle.

Intermittent fasting is not always easy. We need support as much as possible and anything that can make your journey easier. The next chapter will discuss some of the tips that will make your journey smooth and effective.

CHAPTER 8: TIPS FOR MOTIVATION AND SUCCESS

We can do anything we want to if we stick to it long enough.

–Helen Keller

Practice indeed makes perfect. To help you get in the intermittent fasting, I have outlined a few down-to-earth routes and hands-on tips to guide you. Your approach to fasting can mean the difference between success and failure. Consider these tips as guidelines that will help safely implement your preferred fasting regimen.

Start the Day with a Glass of Water

Drink 250 ml of water on an empty stomach first thing in the morning. This will help you boost your energy level and help you digest well throughout the day. Do not drink zesty juice on an empty stomach. It may give you bad gas and a bloated belly.

It is crucial to get enough liquid during the fasting window to survive. You cannot get dehydrated; it will trigger other health problems.

Stay Busy During Your Fasting Window

Avoid staying idle during your fasting window. Staying idle will only keep you thinking about the fast and when it will end. If you are not careful, you might end up breaking your fast before the set time. This is why you should always try to remain busy and productive. Being busy would help you take your mind off the fast. If you are short of activities for the day, you can consider writing your journal, taking a slow walk around the park, reading your favorite book, running some errands, or even going over your goals and why you opt for intermittent fasting in the first place.

Keeping yourself busy at all costs will not only help you forget the fast but also leave you productive. It is an avenue to develop new skills. To help you stay focused on your intermittent fasting goals, you can read up related health, fitness, or weight loss books and write-ups. By just doing one activity or the next, you would be able to distract your mind from redirecting your attention to foods. Also, plan your fasting windows when you're going to be busy doing something.

Maintain Balanced Meals

Having a proper mixture of fiber, carbs, healthy fats, and protein can help shed the extra pounds and fight extreme hunger while fasting. An example of a balanced meal is grilled chicken with mashed potato and sautéed veggies with olive oil. If you want to include fruits in your meals, opt for the ones that come with a low glycemic index, for example, apple, orange, grapefruit, raspberries, avocado, cherry, passion fruit, pears, plums. Choose those fruits which are digested, metabolized, and absorbed slowly. It can help in raising blood glucose slowly. When you have a stable blood sugar level, you can easily avoid all your cravings. Thus, having a balanced meal is the key to shed extra pounds successfully.

Avoid Overeating

Just because you are out of the fasting window doesn't mean you can have a feast. Eating excessively will not only make you feel uncomfortable and bloated, but it can also destroy your goals of weight loss. Overeating can have adverse effects on intermittent fasting. It doesn't matter how much food you have on your plate during the eating window. What is presented on your plate is all that matters.

Break the Fast Steadily and Slowly

After successfully spending many hours without any food, you might think of yourself as a human vacuum that can suck up everything on the plate. However, gulping your food in no time will be of no help to your body. Be careful to break your fast gently. Overeating right after fasting may lead to stomach discomfort. Try to break your fast with a handful of nuts or a small salad to start.

Pay Attention to Your Body

If you are feeling very unwell while fasting, it is important to know when to stop. It is normal to feel fatigued, hungry, and maybe irritable when you fast, but you may want to stop if you feel completely unwell. In order to be safe for your first few times fasting:

1. Keep the duration shorter and work your way up to the desired amount of time.
2. Keep some food on you in case you need to eat something due to low blood sugar or feeling unwell.
3. Remember that you are fasting in order to take care of your body and your health, and it should not make you feel worse.

Engage in Exercise

After following all these tips, favor yourself by exercising. Exercise is the best way to help your body reshape itself. You don't necessarily have to enroll in a gym; you can do all the exercise needed in the comfort of your home. There are a bunch of workouts you can engage yourself in at home that would help in your fasting routine.

Exercising would boost your energy and improve your muscular strength and endurance, thereby leaving you with all the stamina needed for your day's activities. Exercise would also help you burn unnecessary fat. I will provide more information on exercises in Chapter 9.

Keep Track of the Journey

Whether you believe it or not, keeping a food journal can help in maintaining a fasting diet. As you note your emotions, hunger level, weaknesses, cravings, etc., while fasting, you can gauge your progress in a better way. You can also come across some of the trigger points that might make your practice fasting harder for you.

Helpful Tips to Keep You Motivated

Try the following tricks to keep motivated on your intermittent fasting journey.

Make Use of Positive Affirmations

Positive affirmations are very inspiring. They fill us with positive energy and help in clearing away negative thoughts. You can read positive affirmations, listen to them on the internet or recite them loudly. They help in every way. Positive affirmations keep your mind clear and give you the energy to sail through the bad times. They don't take much of your time, and you also don't have to remain dependent on others.

Making use of positive affirmations is a great way to remain motivated. Examples of affirmations:

- "I believe in myself and my ability to succeed. I have hope and certainty about the future."
- "Everything I eat nourishes and strengthens my body and mind."
- "Making small changes is becoming easier. I enjoy the feeling of well-being these changes are giving me."
- "I don't aim for perfection. I accept mistakes and learn from them."
- "I exercise to enjoy a strong, toned body. I love the feeling exercise gives me."

- "I look forward to achieving my ideal weight. This is my goal, and I have the ability to achieve it."

Share Your Goals with Your Family and Friends

Sharing such things with others is always difficult. There is always the fear of being judged on the results. However, there are always some people in everyone's life who don't judge. It can be your partner, siblings, close friends, or parents. Share your goals with them and the problems you are facing. Discuss with them the ways to get out of the problems. They can give you suggestions or at least lend their ears. Even letting it off your chest is also a great relief most of the time.

You will always have an assurance that there are people who really understand your efforts and support you in them. It is unnecessary to disclose your goals to everyone, but sharing them with some of your very close people is always a good idea.

Join a Support Group

It is a cost-effective way to get help. Support groups can emerge as pillars of strength. Many people are suffering from the same problems, going through the same trials and tribulations. Connecting with these people can prove to be a great help if you need moral or mental support. Most of the people in support groups face similar problems, so your problems can be common. You can get the tips that worked for them. Such support groups can be of great help.

Thank God for the Internet; we can now form groups with people of similar interests, even from different continents. Search Facebook or forum websites for fasting groups for women, and you will find many of them. You can then exchange messages, photos, and videos of your progress. That only helps you stay consistent. Share experiences, tips, goals, recipes, survival tactics, and so on. Alone, you can get discouraged and quit, but such a "healthy living family" will not let you fall by the wayside.

Keep the Atmosphere in Your Home Conducive

Most of the time, our surrounding atmosphere also makes our efforts difficult. For instance, if your fridge is full of carbonated beverages, fast food snacks, and munchies, it may be difficult to control the urge to eat. If people in your home are casually eating things all the time, you will start feeling punished and left out. It is important that you explain your goals and make arrangements so that the process gets simpler and not difficult.

Keep Informed

How much do you know about IF? The more you know, the easier it will be for you to go through the process. Read blogs and watch videos to understand what other women have to say about fasting. This will also help you keep your expectations realistic. When it comes to weight loss, women can be impatient. A few days on a diet, and you're already in front of the mirror looking for changes. Don't worry; we've all been there!

You know by now that IF is a way to lose weight fast, but how fast is fast? Getting the right information, especially from those who have gone through the same process already, will let you know what to expect, and you'll be better prepared to deal with any issues that may arise.

***

Chapter Summary

- One of the best decisions you can make during a fast is to drink water. It will keep your body hydrated, and taking water first tithing in the morning or before meals can significantly reduce appetite.

- If you have never tried it before, there is no way you start fasting and go for a whole 48 hours without a meal. For beginners, you can start by having your food at 8 pm, for example, and having nothing again until 8 am the next day. It will be easier since sleep is incorporated into your fasting window.

- Healthy meals should be your priority. They will help you get the required nutrients, which will give you more energy during the fasting period.

- You should not force food hurriedly into your stomach after going long without food, or you might hurt yourself and experience stomach distress. Take it slow when you break your fast. Eat light meals in small portions first when you break your fast. Wait for half an hour or so for your stomach to get used to the presence of food again before continuing with a normal-sized meal.

- When you are on intermittent fasting and not busy, you will be thinking about food, making you break your fast before the stipulated time. You can keep yourself busy by running various errands. Also, plan your fasting windows when you are usually busy during the day, like working at your job or at home.

- You can do mild exercises at home. You will build your muscle strength by exercising, and your body fat will burn faster.

- Practice positive affirmations and share your intermittent fasting goals with your family to keep yourself motivated. Support groups can also emerge as pillars of strength.

Many may wonder if it's safe to exercise during an intermittent fast. With the body depleted of nutrients during a fast after all, would it be wise to put it through any more strain than it is already under? Let's find out in the next chapter.

CHAPTER 9: IF AND EXERCISES

Physical fitness is not only one of the most important keys to a healthy body, it is the basis of dynamic and creative intellectual activity.

–John F. Kennedy

Can I excercise while fasting? All kinds of excercise are encouraged, especially in fasted state. However, some factors need to be considered before combining the two. First, the type of fasting regimen should be considered alongside the individual's physical, mental, and psychological health. Women with existing medical conditions should not combine fasting with exercises before being advised by a medical expert. So, while it is safe to practice intermittent fasting and include exercise if you are an already active person, doing so is not suitable for everyone.

First of all, your metabolism can be negatively impacted if you exercise and fast for long periods. For example, if you exercise daily while fasting daily for more than a month, your metabolic rate can begin to slow down. So, while it may sound like a quick way to reap the benefits of your limited calorie intake, moderation is crucial. Combining the two can trigger a higher rate of breaking down glycogen and body fat. This means that you burn fat at an accelerated rate. Also, when you combine these two, your growth (HGH) hormones are boosted. This results in improved bone density. HGH stimulates the production of collagen, one of the most important building elements of the human body. Because it is the most abundant protein in the body, it also plays a significant role in aging interconnective tissues and muscles. Growth hormone and collagen levels decline as you age. However, increasing your body's HGH content will stimulate collagen formation, resulting in increased muscle growth while strengthening tendons. This is also a quick way to trigger autophagy keeping brain cells and tissues strong, making you feel and look younger.

Did you know that at the age of 40, you may lose about one pound of muscle every year? Once a person reaches the age of 30, they begin to lose muscle mass naturally, and this loss accelerates with time. As a result, your body weakens, and your muscles lose strength, leaving you less flexible and more prone to injury. Furthermore, when you lose muscle, you usually stay the same weight because you gain fat instead, and if you want to lose weight while keeping your body toned, you should combine intermittent fasting with strength workouts.

Exercise is Even Better After 50

Cardiovascular exercise is great for the heart and lungs. It improves oxygen delivery to specific parts of your body, reduces stress, improves sleep, burns fat, and improves sex drive. Some of the more common cardio exercises are running, brisk walking, and swimming. In the gym, machines such as the elliptical, treadmill, and Stairmaster are used to help with cardio. Some people are satisfied and feel like they've done enough after 20 minutes on the treadmill, but if you want to continue to be strong and independent as you grow older, you need to consider adding strength training to your workouts. After 50, strength training for a woman is no longer about six-pack abs, building biceps, or vanity muscles. Instead, it has switched to maintaining a healthy and strong body less prone to injury and illness.

Women over 50 who engage in strength training for 20 to 30 minutes couple of times a week can reap the following benefits:

- **Reduces body fat:** Accumulating excess body fat is not healthy for any woman at any age. To prevent many of the diseases associated with aging, it is important to maintain a healthy body weight by burning excess fat.
- **Build bone density:** With stronger bones, accidental falls are less likely to result in broken limbs or a visit to the emergency room.
- **Build muscle mass:** Although you are not likely to be the next champion bodybuilder, strength training will make you an overall more toned and stronger woman who will

carry herself with ease, push your lawnmower, lift your groceries, and perform all other tasks that require you to exert some strength.

- **Lessen risk of chronic diseases:** In addition to keeping chronic diseases away, strength training can also reduce symptoms of some diseases you may have, such as back pain, obesity, arthritis, osteoporosis, and diabetes. Of course, the type of exercises you do if you have any chronic disease should be recommended by your doctor.
- **Boost mental health:** A loss of self-confidence and depression are some psychological issues that come along with aging. Women who keep themselves fit with exercises tend to be generally more self-assured and are less likely to develop depression.

Strength Training Exercises for Women Over 50

These nine strength training exercises you can do right in the comfort of your home. All you need is a mat, a chair, and some hand weights of about 3-8 pounds, for example, dumbbells or any weights from home like plastic bottles with water. Resistance bands can also be used instead of weights. As you get stronger, you can increase the weight. Take a minute to rest before switching between each exercise. Ensure that you move slowly through the exercises, breathe properly, and focus on maintaining the right form. If you start to feel lightheaded or dizzy during your routines, especially if you are performing the exercise during your fasting window, stop immediately.

Aim for 10-15 reps of each exercise and three sets of each (rest for 1-2 minutes between sets).

Do the strength training workouts 2-3 times each week (with at least 1-2 rest days in between them).

Move your body on all other days when possible. I cover how to do so in the upcoming section.

Squat to Chair

This exercise is great for improving your bone health. Many age-related bone fractures and falls in women involve the pelvis, so this exercise will target and strengthen your pelvic bone and the surrounding muscles.

To perform this:

1. Stand fully upright in front of a chair as if you are ready to sit and spread your feet shoulder-width apart.
2. Extend your arms in front of you and keep them that way throughout the movement.
3. Bend your knees and slowly lower your hips as if you want to sit on the chair, but don't sit. When your butt touches the chair slightly, press into your heels to get back your initial standing position. Repeat that about 10 to 15 times.

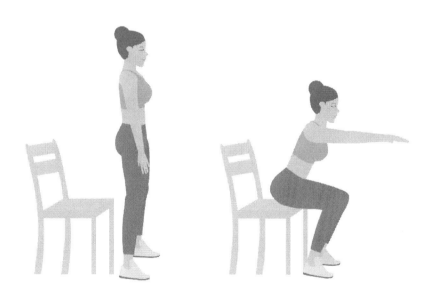

Forearm Plank

This exercise targets your core and shoulders. Here's how to do it:

1. Get into a push-up position, but with your arms bent at the elbows such that your forearm is supporting your weight.

2. Keep your body off the mat or floor and keep your back straight at all times. Don't raise or drop your hips. This will engage your core. Hold the position for 30 seconds, and then drop to your knees. Repeat 3 times.

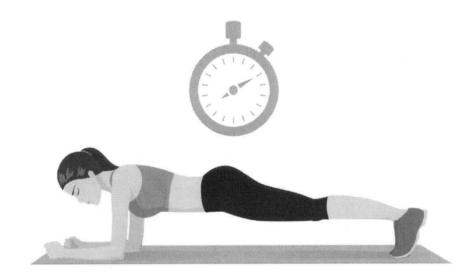

Modified Push-Ups

This routine targets your arms, shoulders, and core. How's how to do it:

1. Kneel on your mat. Place your hands on the mat below your shoulders and let your knees be behind your hips so that your back is straight and long.

2. Tuck your toes under and tighten your abdominal muscles. Gradually bend your elbows as you lower your chest toward the floor.

3. Push back on your arms to press your chest back to your earlier position. Repeat as many times as is comfortable.

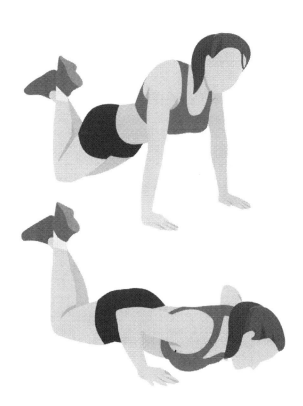

Bird Dog

When done correctly, this exercise can strengthen the muscles of your posterior chain as it targets your back and core. It may seem easy at first, but it can be a bit tricky.

To do this correctly:

1. Go on all fours on your mat.

2. Tighten your abdominal muscles and shift your weight to your right knee and left hand. Slowly extend your right hand in front of you and your left leg behind you. Ensure that both your hands and legs are extended as far as possible and stay in that position for about 5 seconds.

3. Return to your starting position. This is one repetition. Switch to your left knee and right hand and repeat the movement. Alternate between both sides for 20 repetitions.

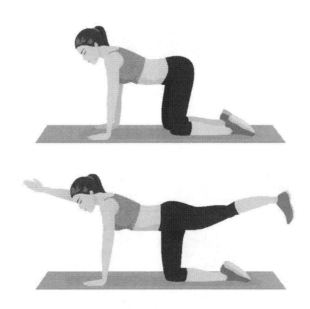

Shoulder Overhead Press

This targets your biceps, shoulders, and back. To perform this move:

1. With dumbbells in both hands, stand and spread your feet shoulder-width apart.

2. Bring the dumbbells up to the sides of your head and tighten your abdominal muscles.

3. Slowly press the dumbbells up until your arms are straight above your head. Slowly return to the first position. Repeat 10 times. You can also do this exercise while sitting.

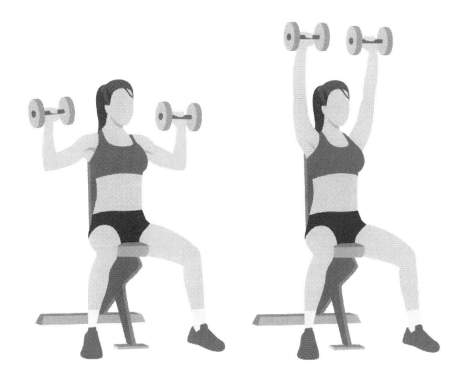

Standing Calf Raise

This exercise improves the mobility of your lower legs and feet and also improves your stability. Here's how to perform it.

1. Stand with your feet flat on the floor, hip-width apart, with your toes facing forward. Use the back of a chair for balance.

2. Raise yourself as high as you can onto the balls of your feet. At the top, squeeze your calf muscles even harder.

3. Slowly and steadily lower your heels back down after a brief pause. If you need extra resistance, you can add extra weight to your hand.

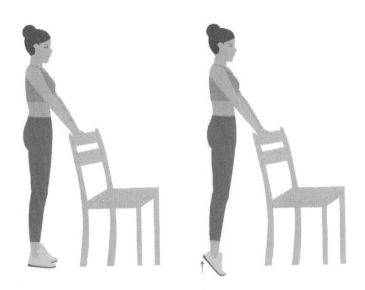

Hamstring Bridge

This move targets your glutes, quads, and hamstrings. To do this:

1. Lie down on your back with your knees bent and your feet on the ground. Throughout the exercise, keep your knees and feet hip-width apart, your toes facing forward, and your ankles just below your knees.

2. With your hands facing down, stretch your arms straight beside your torso. Lift your hips off the mat by pressing through your heels. Squeeze your buttocks together and contract your hamstrings. Pause for 20 to 40 seconds at the top of the bridge position. Return your hips to the ground.

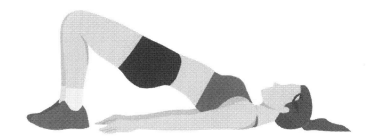

Bent-Over Row

This targets your back muscles and spine. To do this:

1. Hold dumbbells in both hands and stand behind a sturdy object (for example, a chair).

2. Bend forward and rest your head on the chosen object.

3. Relax your neck and slightly bend your knees.

4. With both palms facing each other, pull the dumbbells to touch your ribs.

5. Hold the position for about 2 to 5 seconds and slowly return to the starting position. Repeat 10 to 15 times.

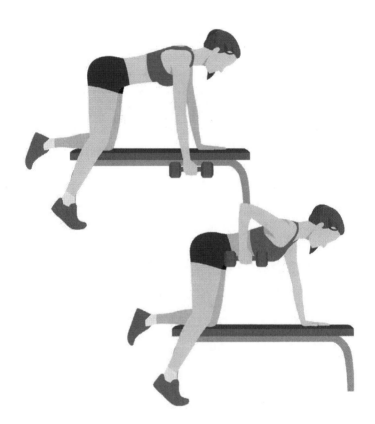

Basic Ab

This exercise can strengthen and tighten the abdominal muscles bringing them inward toward your spine.

To perform this:

1. Lay on your back on the floor, bend your knees. Put your hands behind your head or across your chest while bending your legs. Some say crossing your arms over your chest helps prevent neck yanking. If your neck feels tense, cradle your head with one hand. If you put your hands behind your head, they should gently cradle it. Your goal is to maintain your neck supported as your abs work.

2. To prepare for the action, pull your belly button towards your spine.

3. Slowly contract your abdominals, lifting your shoulder blades off the floor by several inches.

4. As you rise, exhale and keep your neck straight and your chin high. Consider holding a tennis ball beneath your chin. That's the angle you want your chin to be at the entire time.

5. Hold for a few seconds at the apex of the action, breathing constantly.

6. Slowly lower yourself back down, but don't completely relax.

7. Repeat for 15 to 20 reps, perfecting your form each time.

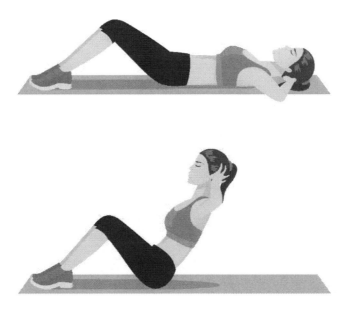

Include Moving Your Body in Your Daily Routine

You do not have to hit the gym or plan a time dedicated to working out. You can make exercise part of your daily routine to always get the proper amount of body movement, whether or not it is time for exercise.

Here are a few tips on including exercises in your daily routine.

- Take the stairs (within reason) instead of using the elevator. You don't want to go up a ten-story building using the stairs! If you have a long way to go up or down, take the stairs a couple of flights and complete your trip with the elevator.

- Find a sporting activity that you thoroughly enjoy and do it as often as is convenient. When you're doing something you enjoy, you'll hardly think of it as exercise, and you're likely to stay committed.

- If you are at work, instead of sending emails or text messages to coworkers, walk up to them and talk to them face to face.

- If possible, convert your one-on-one meetings to walking meetings. Hold the meeting while taking a stroll outside.

- Stop a block or two from your destination and walk the rest of the way. Make walking your preferred mode of transportation.

- Take your dog for walks daily. If you don't have a dog, adopt one. It might seem that you are merely walking your dog, but you are exercising your muscles.

- Take brisk walks as often as possible. Remember to put on comfortable shoes when walking briskly. You can bring your walking shoes with you to make it easy for you to change into them.

- A bit of time gardening, housework (vigorous vacuuming, we might say), walking the children to school will ensure we keep sufficiently on the move.

It will not be the end of the world if you do not find time to engage in any physical activity one day. Furthermore, your body needs a day or two of relaxation during the week. The necessity of resting and recovery will be discussed further.

The Importance of Good Sleep

There are other factors that affect insulin and weight loss, such as sleep deprivation and the stress/cortisol effect. They have to be addressed not with diet but with proper sleep hygiene, meditation, prayer, exercise, social connectivity, or massage therapy. There will be some factors more important than others for each of us. For some, sugars may be the main pathway to obesity; for others, it will be chronic sleep deprivation; for yet others, it will be excessive refined grains; for others, it will be meal timing.

In addition to exercise, sleep is critical for your health. It is the time your body needs to fully recover and do the repair work. If you want good health, you can't ignore sleep. You must give yourself ample time to rest and recover.

To stay healthy and fit, it is important that you don't compromise on your sleep time. It is during your sleep that most essential fat-burning hormones are produced. Your body can repair the damage incurred during the day during your sleep.

One of the biggest side-effects is also problems with sleeping. Sleep apnea is a reality known to most people facing obesity. However, combining intermittent fasting and exercise can help you get good sleep.

You must sleep for 7-8 hours every day. Our bodies do a lot of repair and maintenance work during sleep, and hence, proper sleep is vital. You must also not try to push your body harder beyond the physical limits. A lot of muscles get damaged during exercise, which need time to regenerate. If you don't give them the time, your progress will always be slow and erratic.

The production of IGF-1 (Insulin-like Growth Factor-1) is higher when you are asleep. Because it is a repair hormone, its production is generally at its peak during your sleep. You can boost production by sleeping for optimum hours. The same goes for stress. The higher the levels of stress hormone in your blood, the lower the production of other hormones will put the body in an energy conservation mode. Leading a healthy and positive lifestyle can boost the production of IGF-1 and lower the stress hormone.

Not getting enough sleep can affect your entire day and cause stress to build up.

Sleep deprivation also stimulates overeating and weight gain by increasing the synthesis of the hunger hormone ghrelin.

Here are quick tips on how to improve your sleep hygiene.

- Caffeine and caffeine-based products should be avoided or used in moderation because they disrupt our sleep cycle. Caffeine's effects might persist up to 6 hours after consumption.

- Maintain a sleep schedule. A healthy adult needs at least seven hours of sleep. Most people can attain this aim in eight hours or less.

- Make your room comfortable for sleeping. This often indicates dark, cool, and quiet. Light exposure may make it difficult to fall asleep. Avoid lengthy screen time before bedtime. Use room-darkening shades, earplugs, fans, or other gadgets to create a comfortable setting.

- Taking a relaxing bath or using relaxation techniques like meditation before bedtime may help you sleep better.

- Avoid or limit daytime naps. Long day naps might disrupt night sleep. If you must nap, keep it to 30 minutes and avoid napping late in the day.

- Regular exercise can help you sleep better.

***

Chapter Summary

- Pair your fasting windows with physical activities to get rid of unwanted pounds faster

- Try to have 2-3 strength workouts a week and try to move your body in other ways every other day

- Plan physical activities at the end of the fasting window if possible.

- Give your body the required rest. Do not push it beyond limits. Try to sleep for 7 to 8 hours.

CHAPTER 10: FREQUENTLY ASKED QUESTIONS

To be able to ask a question clearly is two-thirds of the way to getting it answered.

–John Ruskin, an English writer

Intermittent fasting is becoming wildly popular nowadays because of its effects on weight loss and the other health benefits it provides. Because of its popularity, there is a lot of information in circulation.

What to believe and what not to believe becomes difficult in such circumstances. Moreover, if you haven't looked into fasting before, it's natural to have questions.

Well, here are the answers to some common questions that arise in the minds of those who are looking into intermittent fasting for the first time. Now, these answers will give you a different perspective and help you unlearn some misinformation you may have picked up throughout your life. Read along for a sea of information about intermittent fasting that will help bust the myths floating around.

Is it safe for anyone to try intermittent fasting?

Intermittent fasting is not advised for nursing mothers or pregnant women, adolescents/children, underweight people, the sick, or others with a history of disordered eating. Certain individuals on medication can benefit from three regular meals a day after fast.

Additionally, it has been shown that intermittent fasting causes overall tiredness and hunger pains in its practitioners. Certain individuals will find this so destructive that it may begin to impact their way of life; they may feel alone due to being unable to participate in social activities that include food during fasts.

Is it normal for my head to hurt when I fast?

Headache during fasting is a phenomenon that occurs occasionally. Although, in most cases, it disappears after the first few days. It appears that scientific studies have not yet reached any definitive conclusion. However, some associate it with a low blood sugar level or with caffeine withdrawal syndrome. Also, the likelihood of headaches increases with the fast duration and with the individual tendency to suffer it.

A sensible recommendation would be to start small, give the body some time to habituate, and, if the headache persists, discontinue intermittent fasting, or consult a doctor. If you suspect that caffeine may have something to do with it, stick to the same habits while fasting. Remember that you can have tea or coffee alone if they do not contain calories in sugar, milk, or other additives.

What do I do if I do not see results?

It is most likely that you didn't take calorie/energy intake into account, and you overate in your eating window. Then you should try to track your calories to ensure a modest deficit. I like the My Fitness Pal app, where you can enter your current and your goal weight, and the app will calculate your calorie and nutrient goals. Other apps, such as Lose It, FatSecret, LifeSum, Cronometer, can help you count your calorie intake too.

To calculate calories, you can also use this site: https://www.thecalculatorsite.com/

Go to the health section and select the BMR calculator to find out your daily calorie requirements.

You will notice that your selected activity level plays a major role in your calorie requirements. And if you do something physical, you can eat much more.

For a female of 50 years with a height of 5.3 feet and weight of 175 pounds, maintenance calories per day will be:

Activity level	Maintenance calories per day
Sedentary (little or no exercise)	1,670
Lightly active (light exercise or sports 1-3 days per week)	1,914
Moderately active (moderate exercise or sports 3-5 days per week)	2,158
Highly active (hard exercise or sports 6-7 days per week)	2,401
Super athletic (very hard exercise or sports and a physical job)	2,645

For healthy weight loss, the calorie deficit has to be modest, not severe. So, to reach a calorie deficit for healthy weight loss, aim for not more than 20% calorie reduction from nutrition. And if you want an even bigger calorie deficit, create it via exercise. Here, resistance training can help you the most because it will also help fight aging-related muscle loss.

Can you lose weight without doing any exercise?

Absolutely. Do I recommend it? Absolutely not. The reason to move is to burn calories, feel good, and build self-esteem. You can not exercise your way out of a bad diet. If you had one cookie, you have to walk 4 miles; if you eat one supersize meal, you need to run 4 miles a day for a week to burn it off. And if you eat it every day, you have to run a marathon every day just to keep up.

In order to avoid muscle loss, up your protein and do resistance training. You should mix IF methods in order to avoid your body getting used to it and to burn more fat.

How can IF help me to lose weight and go on the path of becoming healthy?

I suggest easing into fasting, perhaps something simple like 16:8. Then migrate to 18:6, 20:4, 22:2, or even OMAD (one meal a day).

What you eat in your feeding window is up to you, but since losing weight is your stated goal, ensure you eat as healthy as possible and make sure it's a modest deficit. Whether you're ok with the word "calorie" or prefer "energy" or even "food portion," the message is the same: you must eat less than you need per day to lose weight.

Most people find that easy when fasting, but not everyone. I, for one, have to track to ensure a deficit; I inherently tend to overeat despite fasting, so I track everything. If you don't need to and you lose weight effortlessly once you start fasting, congrats—you're a natural.

I'm currently doing 16:8. My question is, should I be doing this every day?

The longer you go, the deeper your body goes into fat-burning mode. You are replacing your yucky cells with new good, fresh, healthy cells. My opinion only is that no one should fast every day. Reason being 90% or more of us fast in a calorie deficit, and any long-term calorie deficit results in a drop in metabolism and muscle loss. I haven't yet seen a study beyond eight weeks where this wasn't demonstrated.

Therefore, it's in our best interest to vary our fasts constantly, but be careful not to equate going longer and longer with "varying." We need days off. I typically take Mondays off, not eating after supper Sunday through lunch on Tuesday.

Then, I alternate 18:6 or 20:4 with days off. You can do 12:12 if you like. Fasting days are a pretty good deficit (about 1500 cals), but I eat at maintenance on 12:12 days (2100 cals). I lost 70lbs over two years on that plan.

Can I drink something during the fast?

Of course, you can drink liquids as long as they are low or no-calorie beverages. Non-caloric liquids are liquids that do not contain any calories. Water, black tea, black coffee, organic tea, bone broth, unsweetened juices, and some soups are all non-caloric liquids.

In fact, you should drink plenty of liquids during your fast since fasting causes dehydration. Liquids also help in managing hunger by suppressing appetite.

Our goals during fasting are to control hunger and keep the body hydrated. Therefore, you can and should drink liquids.

Only make certain that you are not adding sugar to your coffee, tea, and juices. If you add sugar, it just defeats the purpose of fasting. We are fasting to burn the glycogen and fat stores; therefore, added sugar defeats the purpose, making fasting a waste of time.

Can I work out while fasting?

Yes, you can work out, and I would say you should. It will aid weight loss, burn more fat, help in muscle gain, and balance hormones. Opt for low-intensity workouts. We don't want to stress our bodies. An hour of restorative yoga, walking, jogging, and gardening are some of the exercises you could do. They will also reduce the stress and anxiety that come with menopause. Don't push yourself while exercising. Go slow and keep the duration short. If you start feeling dizzy, take a break. Stop exercising if you feel pressure or pain in the chest, an irregular heartbeat, shortness of breath, nausea, or pain in your jaw, left arm, or shoulder. Lie down if you face any of these symptoms and call for medical help. Plan your workout at the end of the fasting window if possible.

Chapter Summary

- Intermittent fasting is not advised for nursing mothers or pregnant women, adolescents/children, underweight people, the sick, or others with a history of disordered eating.

- It is normal to experience headaches once you begin your intermittent fasting. If you experience such symptoms, start small, give the body some time to habituate, and, if the headache persists, discontinue intermittent fasting, or consult a doctor.

- You should always try to track your calories to ensure a modest deficit. Use apps like My Fitness Pal or any app of your choice.

- Our goals during fasting are to control hunger and keep the body hydrated. Therefore, you can and should drink liquids as long as they are low or no-calorie beverages.

- It is also important to pair your intermittent fasting with exercise. However, you should start with low-intensity workouts. For example, jogging or gardening as your body gets used to exercising. If possible, it would be great if you plan your workouts at the end of the fasting window.

WOULD YOU DO ME A SMALL FOVOR?

Thank you for reading this book. I hope you'll use what you've learned to look, feel and live better than you ever have before.

I have a small favor to ask.

Would you mind taking a minute to write a blurb on Amazon about this book? I check all my reviews and love to get honest feedback. That's the real pay for my work – knowing that I'm helping people.

Thanks again, and I really look forward to reading your feedback!

To post your review scan with your camera:

CONCLUSION

Intermittent fasting is not a fad diet but a way of life—a lifestyle.

A lifestyle cannot be right or wrong.

Fasting has been around for as many years as the evolution of humans. Most of the cultures and religions in the world encourage fasting for various reasons.

But fasting for health is something that has started in recent years and has caught the fancy of many people, both young and old, all across the world.

The health benefits of intermittent fasting are many, as we have discussed throughout this book, especially for women in their 40s and 50s, when they find it difficult to lose weight and face threats from many diseases due to the hormonal changes happening in their bodies.

But every woman is unique. And her experience of passing through menopause is also unique. Some women may not experience any symptoms, and menopause may seem a smooth ride for them. While for some others, the symptoms may be so severe that it may hamper their way of life.

In such a scenario, all that can be said is intermittent fasting is a lifestyle change and not a medical treatment. You should give it a try after consulting your doctor and under their watchful supervision. Thereafter, let your body adjust to the fasting way of life for a few days and observe the changes in your physical and mental wellbeing. If you see any positive effects, continue the intermittent fast as per your capabilities. But if you experience the side effects of intermittent fasting, make changes to your fasting schedule as is appropriate to eliminate the side effects. Listen to your body and observe the changes happening to it.

Also, if you have long-lasting adverse effects from intermittent fasting, your body may be rejecting it.

Don't keep up with intermittent fasting if it makes you miserable.

While this manner of eating has been linked to health benefits, there are many more ways to improve your health without fasting.

Maintaining a healthy diet, getting enough sleep, exercising regularly, and managing stress are far more important for overall health.

What to expect? Weight loss amount varies from person to person. Changing fasting protocol can help to break when you hit plateau.

I hope this book has added value to your life. I have tried to cover all about intermittent fasting and its effect for women above 50 years of age in as much detail as possible, without being overly preachy. Do send in your feedback for the book. I am looking forward to hearing from you!

REFERENCES

Boost, J. (2021, December). INTERMITTENT FASTING FOR WOMEN OVER 50: The Ultimate Beginner's Guide with Tips & Tricks to Get Rid of Extra Weight, Feel Good About Yourself Again and Have Fun with Your New Lifestyle. Independently published. ASIN: B09P3XB6FN.

Che, T., Yan, C., Tian, D., Zhang, X., Liu, X., & Wu, Z. (2021). Time-restricted feeding improves blood glucose and insulin sensitivity in overweight patients with type 2 diabetes: a randomised controlled trial. *Nutrition & Metabolism, 18*(1). https://doi.org/10.1186/s12986-021-00613-9.

Clark, J. (2021, October). Intermittent Fasting for Women Over 50 : The Simple Formula for Losing Weight, Promoting Longevity, and Feeling Great After 50: Master All Secrets of Fasting to Unlock Metabolism and Detox Your Body. Independently published. ASIN: B09JJ7FPZV.

Eenfeldt, J. (2022, January). Intermittent Fasting for Women Over 50: The Guide to Lose Weight without Hunger Pangs and Increase your Energy, 8 Techniques that Led Me to Success +101 Mouth-Watering Recipes and a 14-Day Eating Plan. Independently published. ASIN: B09R3C4W1F.

Francis, N. (2020). The role of intermittent fasting in brain health. *Alzheimer's & Dementia, 16*(S10). https://doi.org/10.1002/alz.0439.

Fung, D. J. (2018, March). Why Fasting Succeeds Where Caloric Restriction Fails. Medium. Retrieved from https://betterhumans.pub/why-caloric-restriction-fails-part-2-ec0c0c337649.

Fung, J. (September, 2018). How fasting affects your physiology and hormones. Diet Doctor. Retrieved from https://www.dietdoctor.com/fasting-affects-physiology-hormones.

Gill, A. (2021, May). Intermittent Fasting For Women Over 50: Guide to Longer and Healthier Life – Boost Your Metabolism and Accelerate Weight Loss, Detox and Rejuvenate Your Body with 150+ recipes and 30 days meal plan. Independently published. ASIN: B09HHVPVTR.

Gunnars, K. (2020, April). Intermittent Fasting 101: The Ultimate Beginner's Guide. Healthline. Retrieved from https://www.healthline.com/nutrition/intermittent-fasting-guide.

Keenan, S., Cooke, M. B., & Belski, R. (2020). The Effects of Intermittent Fasting Combined with Resistance Training on Lean Body Mass: A Systematic Review of Human Studies. *Nutrients, 12*(8), 2349. https://doi.org/10.3390/nu12082349.

Kim, S. H., & Park, M. J. (2017). Effects of growth hormone on glucose metabolism and insulin resistance in human. *Annals of Pediatric Endocrinology & Metabolism, 22*(3), 145–152. https://doi.org/10.6065/apem.2017.22.3.14.

Land, S. (2018, June 25). How Much Protein to Eat While Intermittent Fasting. Siim Land Blog. Retrieved from https://siimland.com/how-much-protein-to-eat-while-intermittent-fasting/.

Mayo Clinic Staff. (2020, November 10). Can you boost your metabolism? Mayo Clinic. Retrieved from https://www.mayoclinic.org/healthy-lifestyle/weight-loss/in-depth/metabolism/art-20046508.

McIntosh, J. (2020, January 24). Ketosis: Symptoms, diet, and more. Medical News Today. Retrieved from https://www.medicalnewstoday.com/articles/180858.

Meixner, M. (2018, October 2). Does Eating Late at Night Cause Weight Gain? Healthline. Retrieved from https://www.healthline.com/nutrition/eating-at-night.

Morgan, L. (2021, August). Intermittent Fasting for Women Over 50: Start To Lose Weight, Delay Aging And Boost Your Energy With Quick, Easy and Healthy Recipes To Reset Your Metabolism. Exercises and 14 Days Meal Plan Included. Independently published. ASIN: B09CRY92XK.

Pesta, D. H., & Samuel, V. T. (2014). A high-protein diet for reducing body fat: mechanisms and possible caveats. *Nutrition & Metabolism, 11*(1), 53. https://doi.org/10.1186/1743-7075-11-53.

Petre, A. (2019, June). Does "Calories in vs. Calories out" Really Matter? Healthline. Retrieved from https://www.healthline.com/nutrition/calories-in-calories-out.

West, H. (2016, November). Does Intermittent Fasting Boost Your Metabolism? Healthline. Retrieved from https://www.healthline.com/nutrition/intermittent-fasting-metabolism.

Wheeler, H. L. (2022, February). Intermittent Fasting for Women Over 50: Easy Step-by-Step Science-Based Guide to Lose Weight, Increase your Energy and Delay Aging. 30 Days Meal Plan and 130 Recipes Included. Independently published. ASIN: B09SXZKRVW.

Wildman, K. (2021, August). Intermittent Fasting for Women Over 50: A Perfect Guide to Losing Weight, Reset Your Metabolism, Boost Your Energy and Eating Healthy with 60+ Recipes and 21 Days Meal Plan. Independently published. ASIN: B09DL4SLPX.

Why You Shouldn't Fear Fasting with Dr. Jason Fung and Jimmy Moore (2016, December). Dave Asprey. https://daveasprey.com/why-you-shouldnt-fear-fasting-with-dr-jason-fung-and-jimmy-moore/

Image Credit: oldwayspt.org, shutterstock.com

ATKINS DIET FOR BUSY WOMEN

Look and Feel Better by Eating Satisfying Foods You Really Enjoy

Nathalie Seaton

SPECIAL BONUS!

Want This Bonus book for FREE?

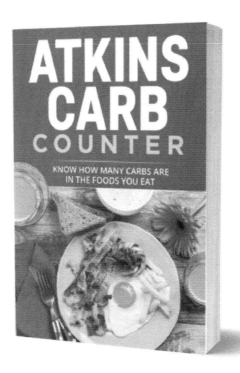

Get FREE unlimited access to it and all of my new books by joining the Fan Base!

SCAN W/ YOUR CAMERA TO JOIN!

INTRODUCTION

The Atkins Diet has been tried and tested for decades, with proven results. Although it is a popular celebrity diet, it was designed to suit the needs and budget of everyone. The Atkins Diet was created to help people eat everyday whole foods more beneficially. You will probably already have a lot of the approved diet foods in your pantry because you eat normal everyday foods on the Atkins Diet. Because you eat regular foods that you can buy at any grocery store, the diet is easily adapted to fit into your lifestyle. You will look and feel better while still eating the satisfying foods you really enjoy.

Dieting the Atkins way means only having to make some adjustments to your eating habits, and not your entire way of life. Most other diets make you slash your portion size, which leaves you feeling hungry and more inclined to cheat or give up. Although the Atkins Diet recommends portion control, it is in the sense that you eat until you're full and don't overeat or exceed your recommended daily carbohydrate allowance.

On the Atkins Diet, there is no calorie counting, on again or off again days, or fasting intervals. You eat three square meals a day with room for two light snacks in between. You won't feel hungry during the day. Because you are limiting your carb intake and not overeating, your body burns fat as its fuel source, thus leaving you feeling more alive, energized, and alert. You will also look amazing and have a lot more confidence.

There are many benefits to living the Atkins way. One of which ensures that those extra pounds you lose stay off for good. An Atkins lifestyle will also improve the quality of your life and health. Once you have been on the diet for a couple of weeks, you will realize just how easy it is to slip into the Atkins way of life.

As the Atkins Diet means making healthier choices from the foods you love, if you have family, there is no need to make two separate meals each mealtime. Your family can also enjoy and benefit from the delicious healthy meals you make on this diet.

Women face many body change challenges throughout their life. We go through puberty, pregnancy, menopause, and the many other growing pains in between. While all this is happening, we still have to deal with our everyday lives. What is so great about the Atkins Diet is that it can be adjusted and adapted to fit into our busy lifestyles! We don't have to make drastic changes to fit our lifestyle into it. No matter if you are pregnant, breastfeeding, raising children, or menopausal, the Atkins Diet can work for you.

There is one thing that can put a person off the Atkins Diet, especially a person with an already hectic life. At first glance, the diet appears a little complex and not everyone has the time to browse through websites and books with conflicting information. I know this firsthand from when I started on the Atkins diet some years ago as a busy woman with a family, an executive job, and fast heading towards middle age. There were several times I wanted to quit because I did not have the time to dig for the information I needed, especially in the first two weeks of the diet when your body is adjusting to the limited carb intake and you are trying to overcome your cravings.

I have had a lot of success on the Atkins Diet and feel that my family has also benefited from my healthier and carb-conscious choices. I started having children late in life and struggled to lose a lot of the weight I had gained with my firstborn. That is when I started the Atkins Diet. To be honest, it was a battle for me in the beginning and it did not need to be; this inspired me to write this book.

I have written *Atkins Diet for Busy Women* to help you save time getting started on the Atkins Diet plan. The book breaks the Atkins Diet into easy to follow sections. There is a comprehensive list of approved foods and their net carb value per portion size per phase. There is also a comprehensive list of foods to avoid.

To make your meal planning easier, I have included a seven-day meal plan for Phase 1 and Phase 2 to get you started. There are a few exercise ideas to add to the benefits of your healthier lifestyle along with what common mistakes to avoid when getting started and step-by-step delicious low-carb recipes to try. By the end of this book, you will know exactly how the Atkins Diet works and be well on your way to achieving your weight loss goals.

CHAPTER 1: THE ATKINS DIET

Dr. Robert Atkins was a cardiologist who introduced the Atkins diet in the 1960s. He developed this diet because of his growing concerns for the increase of the overweight and obese.

If you eat more carbohydrates than your body can use, it will store the excess carbs as fat. This means you are at greater risk of gaining weight. Carrying excess weight may increase a person's risk of developing diseases such as diabetes or heart disease.

The Atkins Diet plan limits the number of carbohydrates in a diet according to a person's needs while increasing proteins and fats. It is not a diet that needs you to count calories, and it does not limit portion sizes. However, you need to be aware of the number of carbohydrates you are eating per day. Most foods you buy at the store these days come with a nutritional label on it. This makes it easy to keep track of each food item's carbohydrate value.

When the Atkins Diet first came out, they nicknamed it the "steak and eggs diet" because the diet allowed fried eggs and fatty meat cuts. Because of Dr. Atkins' fresh approach to losing weight, his diet plan was, at first, highly criticized. Over the years, thousands of people have successfully lost weight on his diet plan. Not only have they lost weight, but by adopting the Atkin's way of eating as a lifestyle, they have kept the weight off.

Since Dr. Atkins introduced the diet plan, it has been adapted and refined to move with the times and health trends over the decades. In the modern-day era, the diet can adapt to suit any lifestyle, including vegetarians and vegans.

How the Atkins Diet Works

Unlike a lot of other diet plans, the Atkins Diet does not require calorie counting, or on again off again days, and there are no restrictive portion controls. A regular diet that counts calories may still not sufficiently control or limit carbs in the diet. This can cause problems such as feeling flat, tired, and moody because carbs affect blood sugar.

The Atkins Diet requires a person to keep tight control of the carbohydrates they consume during the day. Your body will no longer burn sugar; instead, it will burn fat during the day if you limit the number of carbs you eat. As a result, you will feel more awake, energized, and alert while shedding pounds.

There are three different Atkins plans to choose from; the plan you choose will depend on your weight loss or lifestyle goals. The three Atkins diet plans are:

Atkins 20 Diet Plan

This is the original Atkins diet plan and the most popular one to start with.

- The diet plan is broken into four different phases (Phase 1 to Phase 4), and each phase has a set amount of carbs you can eat per day. As you reach your goal weight and progress to the next phase, you can slowly increase the amount and types of carbs you eat per day.

- In Phase 1, you will eat 20 to 25 grams of carbs per day.

- It is a diet plan for anyone who has more than 40 pounds to lose.

- It is also a good diet for anyone who is either pre-diabetic or diabetic.

- It is for someone who wants to maintain their weight and adapt the diet as a lifestyle. People looking to maintain their weight usually start at Phase 3 or 4 of this plan.

Atkins 40 Diet Plan

This is an Atkins diet plan that has a little more flexibility with the type of carbs you eat and the amount you eat per day.

- On this plan, you will start with 40 grams of carbs per day.

- Your carb intake will increase by 10 grams when you reach your goal weight.

- This diet is ideal for anyone who has fewer than 40 pounds to lose.

- It is ideal for women who are pregnant or breastfeeding (under the strict guidance of a doctor or health care advisor).

- This Atkins diet plan gives you a larger selection of foods you can eat from the start.

Atkins 100 Diet Plan

This plan is for those who are wanting to make the Atkins Diet an everyday part of their healthy eating plans.

- On this plan, you will start with 100 grams of carbs per day.

- Your carb intake and portion controls stay the same.

- This diet is ideal for anyone who wants to maintain their current weight and eat healthier.

- Under the strict guidance of a doctor or health care provider, it can be used by women who are pregnant or breastfeeding.

- This Atkins diet plan allows you the freedom to choose the foods that you want to eat within the given carb limitations.

Please note that these three plans are as they appear on the atkins.com website at the time this book was printed. Some global Atkins websites do not offer or reference these three plans. You may find that these global sites still use the Atkins Diet Phase 1 through 4 for weight loss, weight control maintenance, and lifestyle plans.

Remember to always check with a doctor before starting any new weight loss or lifestyle plans. This is especially important if you have an existing health issue or are pregnant.

What Are the Benefits of the Atkins Diet?

There are many reasons for eating a low-carbohydrate diet. Here are some major benefits:

- Your body burns fat instead of carbohydrates for energy, resulting in the loss of excess body fat.

- Cravings of carbohydrate-rich food eventually stop, breaking the cycle of overeating because of carb highs and lows.

- When the cravings stop, you don't feel hungry all the time.

- The Atkins Diet promotes an improved level of HDL (the good cholesterol your body needs).

- You feel more alert as your concentration improves and blood-sugar stabilizes.

- Stable blood sugar levels also improve upon a person's moods, and you will have fewer mood swings.

- You will feel less bloated within a week or two from starting a low-carb diet. This is because carbs encourage the body to retain water.

- As there is no counting calories or a set food plan; you are more likely to find something you can eat on a menu at a restaurant.

- Overall, you will feel more energetic, you will not feel so tired all the time, and you will look and feel great about yourself.

Atkins Results & Inspirational Success Stories

Please note that the names in the stories have been changed.

Pam — 25 years old from California — Lost 20 pounds

Pam had been overweight since going through puberty in her late teens. Through ups and downs in her personal life and having a baby halfway through college, her weight increased. As her weight increased, Pam became more and more insecure and started to grow to dislike herself. The more she disliked her body, the more she would comfort herself with high-carb and sugar-filled foods. Until one day her husband started to follow the Atkins Diet plan. Intrigued by how well her husband was eating and what he could eat, Pam decided to give it a go. That was three years ago. Not only did Pam manage to lose all that weight, but by making some changes to her eating habit and exercising, she has also managed to keep the weight off. She is more confident, has more energy, and looks absolutely stunning. Pam is a busy mom of three, who has easily managed to adapt the Atkins Lifestyle to fit into her way of life.

Desire — 49 years old from Boston — Lost 18 pounds

Up until Desire was 39 years old, she had always been super health-conscious and fit. She had her first baby at the age of 39. She kept up her vigorous exercise routing well into her fourth trimester of pregnancy. During the last month of her pregnancy, her body seemed to pop out and she gained quite a bit of weight. Once her baby was born, the weight kept piling. As a busy new mother, career woman, and wife, she hardly had time to breathe, let alone think about her eating habits. When her son was five years old, he asked her if she had another baby in her belly because it was so big. That is when Desire decided it was time to find a way to lose weight. She needed a diet that was more than an eating plan and one that she could easily fit around her entire family. That is when she found the Atkins Diet. Desiree lost 18 pounds five years ago, and losing those pounds changed her life for the better. Living the Atkins Lifestyle, Desire has managed to keep those pounds at bay. She still enjoys the foods she loves, and by making a few changes for each member of her family to the diet, she keeps her family eating healthy as well.

Jackie — 55 years old from New York — Lost 65 pounds

Jackie struggled to lose weight as she juggled a high-stress job, a messy divorce, and getting used to an empty nest. After her children left home to study or move on with their own lives, Jackie threw herself into her work to fill the void. As she no longer had anyone to cook for, fast foods, TV dinners, or a snack bar became her everyday meals. Being over 50, Jackie was also going through menopause, which added to the weight gain effects of her unhealthy eating habits. After many failed attempts at fad diets, Jackie gave up with her weight until her daughter got engaged to be married. It was not long after that, that Jackie found out she was pre-diabetic and was warned to lose weight. Her health scare and her daughter's upcoming marriage were Jackie's wake-up call. A friend of hers introduced her to the Atkins Diet, and with the support of her family and friends, Jacket lost 65 pounds. That was three years ago and to date Jackie has kept the weight off, she now lives a healthy Atkins Lifestyle and is engaged to be married once again. Her health has improved, she feels more energized and alive than she ever felt before going on the Atkins Diet.

CHAPTER 2: WHERE TO BEGIN

Deciding to change your eating habits to improve your health is the first big step to a healthier lifestyle. Choosing the correct diet is the second step in starting a diet. Most people skip the next few steps and dive right into their diets. There is nothing wrong with being eager to get your diet started and the path to shedding those extra pounds or being healthy. In fact, being eager and excited over changing your eating habits is a good start.

A successful diet means self-preparation and organization. You may know why you need to diet, how you are going to diet, and the foods to eat. But that may not prepare you for the impact it will have on you or your life. Being eager to start the diet will not keep you motivated for too long if you are not fully prepared. This chapter will help you better prepare yourself for getting started on your Atkins Diet journey. It will help you set realistic goals, find challenges you may face, help you understand supplements, and more.

Are There Health Risks?

As with any diet, there are always health risks. This is especially true if you have preexisting health conditions and/or are pregnant, menopausal, or of an advanced age.

The beginning of the Atkins Diet, Phase 1, drastically cuts a person's carb intake and can cause some side effects. Some of the most common side effects experienced on the Atkins Diet are:

- Constipation
- Dizziness
- Fatigue
- Headache
- Weakness

Should any of the symptoms persist or you become concerned, seek immediate medical advice.

If you can stick to the Atkins Diet and get over the first few weeks, the diet can have some positive effects on your health. It may also improve on some serious health conditions which include:

- Cardiovascular disease
- Diabetes
- Improve blood cholesterol
- High blood pressure
- Metabolic syndrome

Adjusting the Atkins Diet During Pregnancy, Breast Feeding, Post Menopause

In pregnancy, and under the careful guidance of your doctor, you can maintain a healthy weight. Any extra pounds you may have gained will be a lot easier to shed when you can eat normally again.

Women who are heading for or going through menopause have to take extra care with what foods they eat. You also have to consider the hormone fluctuations, lack of sleep as your sleep patterns change, loss of muscle mass, and an increase in insulin resistance. Low-carb diets, such as the Atkins Diet, have been shown to be far more effective for weight loss at this time of a woman's life, especially for getting rid of belly fat (Gardner et al., 2007).

As there are risks to any diet, this risk can increase if a woman is pregnant, breastfeeding, or post-menopause. The Atkins websites have some documentation on this, but it is best to seek the advice of a doctor or nutritionist. Trained specialists will adjust and adapt the Atkins diet to suit your individual needs. When you are pregnant, there are certain foods you need to avoid, and this is the same if you are breastfeeding. Although there are general foods to avoid like shellfish, coffee, alcohol, etc., your pregnancy may require extra nutrients or specific dietary requirements.

When a woman is premenopausal, you may require extra nutrients and supplements. These will need to be expertly fit into your diet to ensure proper weight loss and be beneficial to your health. Once again, although following the diet as it is will still be beneficial, to get the most from the Atkins Diet it is best to seek a licensed professional's advice.

Am I Ready to Change My Lifestyle?

One of the big questions you should ask yourself before you jump in and begin dieting is *"Am I ready to change my lifestyle?"* Because that is what you are doing: you are making a change to your lifestyle. One of the big reasons most diets fail is because people see them as a quick fix to losing weight.

The sad reality is that a lot of these fad diets are just a way to shed a few pounds fast. A lot of these diets do offer quick weight loss, but as with everything that seems too good to be true, these diets don't work. They may seem like they are working at first. You may even see results quite fast. But for how long will you keep that weight off? What cost to your health, your well-being, and your pocket did you have to pay?

If you are reading this book, then you have decided it is time to make a more drastic change to your eating habits. With the success rate of the Atkins diet, you have made the right choice. But deciding it is time for a change and finding the right diet is only part of the process of getting ready for a lifestyle change. Another part of the dieting process is accepting that this is not just a diet. It is a lifestyle; you are going to have to make some changes. But with Atkins, the changes are not that drastic.

You need to ask yourself the following questions:

- Why am I wanting to diet?
- What am I trying to accomplish?
- Do I want to lose weight for a special occasion?
- Do I want to lose the extra pounds I have gained recently or over the years?
- Do I want to get healthy?
- Do I want to make sure the pounds I lose stay off for good?
- Am I ready to change my eating habits and commit to a healthier lifestyle?

147

The Atkins Diet is about learning to eat the foods you love the right way. I am not going to lie because there are some foods you will have to do away with. But the good news is there are always healthier alternatives to substitute the foods with.

You just have to commit to making the changes and give them a try. One of the best things about the Atkins diet is that you don't have to turn your life upside down. You choose the foods you want to eat from the acceptable foods list. For the first two weeks, you do have a limited selection, but it is quite a large list of foods on that list.

The diet does not end after the first two weeks. You progress onto the next phase of the diet, which introduces an even wider variety of food choices. As you progress to the maintenance and lifestyle phase, you realize how simple eating healthy actually is. That a few simple changes in what you eat and how you eat it can make a huge difference to your weight and overall health.

For a diet to be successful, you need to commit to it for a lifetime. Otherwise, your weight and health will most likely continue to yo-yo back and forth. Do you really want to put all this effort into losing weight and getting healthy, only to fall back into bad habits? Looking at a diet as something you have to do for a certain length of time is why most people land right back where they started.

Now, ask yourself again, are you ready to commit to a lifestyle change?

Think of it as cleaning out your closet and everything you get rid of, must go for good. You are going to keep all the basics and your favorites, but you are going to shake things up a little and add a few new bits. By the time you have finished your first two weeks on the diet, your body will have already started to adjust to the new routing. After four weeks, you will find that even the way you grocery shop will have changed.

So, if you are ready for a wardrobe change, then it is time to take the next step.

What Are My Goals?

There are no quick fixes or magic potions you can take that will make the pounds dissolve or magically transform you. Now that you are ready to make the change for a healthier, slimmer you, you don't want to stumble at your first hurdle. That first hurdle for most people looking to lose weight is setting realistic goals.

Losing weight too quickly may seem like a good thing but it is not. Not only is it mostly water your body loses, but it is not very good for your health. To burn fat, you need to have a healthy balance of carbohydrates in your body. Not too much that your body will store the excess as fat, but not too little that your body has no energy reserves either.

If you do lose weight too quickly, your body will quickly reach a plateau where your weight loss will slow down or stop altogether. This also becomes a turning point for some people and they just throw in the towel, then revert to their old habits. Then there is the part where you may look good having shed those pounds but you probably don't feel that great. To get there more than likely took a lot out of you physically, mentally, and emotionally.

Stick to the wise words of the tortoise in the story about the tortoise and the hare, "*Slow and steady wins the race.*" A healthy weekly weight loss should be no more than one to two pounds. If you are exercising, you will need to set goals and an achievable routine to accommodate your fitness plan. As with weight loss, set steady achievable goals for yourself that are not going to wear you out and leave you aching.

If you have any pre-existing conditions, concerns, or need a bit of advice, speak to a healthcare professional, nutritionist, or dietician. They will be able to give you your correct BMI and what your ideal weight should be. When you set your overall weight loss goals, this also needs to be realistic. You don't want to get too thin as, once again, you are only going to be playing with your health and well-being.

What Are My Current Commitments?

The above question is more about commitment to your way of life. For example:

- Do you have a family?
    - If you do, you will need to consider what their dietary needs are.
    - How hard will it be to adjust the Atkins eating plan to accommodate them?
    - Don't let this be a stumbling block because it is not that hard to pad carbs for growing children or grown partners. It can even be adjusted to suit the needs of the elderly. Keep in mind that this diet is more about cutting down on carbs and swapping out foods for healthier ones.
- Do you have certain dietary needs?
    - If you have special dietary needs for various reasons, you can work with your health care provider to adjust the Atkins Diet to suit your requirements.
- Do you have any pre-existing conditions?
    - For pre-existing conditions, you should always check with your doctor before starting a new eating plan, no matter what it is.
    - Your doctor will help you or put you in touch with the right person to help you adjust the Atkins Diet to suit your needs.
- Is there anything in your current lifestyle that will stop you from implementing your new lifestyle change?
    - This could be anything from resistance from your family.
    - Pressures at work.
    - Turmoil in your personal life.
    - Financial issues.
    - Once you have these listed down try and work in a plan of how you can overcome these obstacles to get you started on the eating plan. Even if you start off making small changes, you will have made a start.

Do I Need Nutritional Supplements?

Every diet needs the recommended daily dosage of vitamins and antioxidants. Even when a person is on a well-balanced diet, they may not be getting enough of these vital nutrients.

Although it is good practice to take multivitamins or certain supplements, always check with a medical professional first. Some medical conditions may be affected by certain substances in supplements.

There are many different multivitamins on the market. The one you choose will depend on your nutrient needs. Some of the essential nutrients the body needs are:

- **Biotin** — Biotin is sometimes referred to as vitamin H or vitamin B7 and it is vital for good skin, nails, and hair health. It also aids the body in converting some nutrients into energy.

- **Boron** — Although not one of the top essential vitamins, boron plays a role in bone health, testosterone levels, estrogen levels, and it helps the body convert certain minerals and vitamins.

- **Calcium** — Calcium is mainly stored in the teeth and bones as it plays a vital role in maintaining and supporting them. This mineral also plays a part in helping the nervous system distribute messages to and from the brain. It is important for maintaining the fluid movement of the muscles.

- **Chromium** — Your body needs small amounts of chromium to help with insulin sensitivity, protein breakdown, building muscle, and controlling weight.

- **Folate** — Folate is an essential nutrient that aids your body in the production of genetic material, including DNA.

- **Iodine** — Iodine helps the body's metabolism by making thyroid hormones, which are also essential for the development of the brain and bones.

- **Iron** — The lack of iron is a cause of anemia as iron is needed to help oxygenate the blood and produce red blood cells.

- **Magnesium** — Magnesium helps to produce strong healthy bones and DNA, and it helps to keep your blood pressure and blood sugar regulated.

- **Potassium** — Potassium helps the body's muscles and nervous system to function correctly.

- **Selenium** — Selenium has quite a few vital functions in the body, one of which is protecting it from free radicals.

- **Vitamin A** — Vitamin A has a lot to offer the body, including helping the heart, kidneys, and lung function correctly. Beta-carotene is part of the Vitamin A family and it actively helps to keep the immune system healthy, as well as helping with vision.

- **Vitamin B6** — This is a very important vitamin that the body needs to help with various functions such as metabolizing carbohydrates, protein, and fats. It is also needed for the production of neurotransmitters and red blood cells.

- **Vitamin B12** — Vitamin B12 helps the body create DNA for cells and red blood cells, and it keeps the body's nervous system healthy.

- **Vitamin C** — Vitamin C can also be called ascorbic acid. It provides the body with a lot of help with keeping the skin, hair, and nails healthy. It ensures the blood vessels are healthy and aids in the maintenance of good bone health.

- **Vitamin D** — The sun is the most powerful source of vitamin D. But there are many places where there is not a lot of sunlight all year around. A deficiency of vitamin D can lead to a problem called rickets, which is a bone deformity found in children. This vitamin is essential for strong bones and teeth and to help keep the amount of phosphate and calcium in the body regulated.

- **Vitamin E** — Vitamin E is one of the many vitamins that are essential for good skin health. It also helps the body fight off the damaging effects caused by free radicals.

- **Vitamin K** — Vitamin K helps with bone health and blood clotting.

- **Zinc** — Zinc is found in all the cells in the body. This is an essential nutrient that helps the body fight off intruders such as viruses and bacteria. It also helps in the production of genetic materials including DNA.

Keep a Progress Journal

Keeping a progress journal will help you keep track of your weekly weight loss. You can also keep a quick list of your favorite foods and their net carbs. You can document the foods you love, can tolerate, and cannot stand. It is also a great place to keep your favorite recipes and the ones you make on your own.

It is also a safe place to jot down how you are feeling and your exercise regime.

Getting Started With the Atkins Diet

In a previous section of this chapter, you read about setting yourself realistic and attainable goals. Goals that will not affect your health while still leaving you feeling healthy and energetic. Once your goals are set and you have your motivation, you are ready to choose the correct Atkins Diet plan to suit your individual needs.

To choose the correct Atkins Diet plan/phase for you, you need to ask yourself:

- Do you want to lose weight or maintain your weight and eat healthier?
- If so, do you have over forty pounds to lose? If you do, you will need to start with Phase 1 — The Induction Phase.
- If you have less than 40 pounds to lose, look at starting at Phase 2 — The Ongoing Weight Loss plan, referred to as OWL for short.
- If you want to maintain your weight and want to live the "Atkins Lifestyle," look at starting at Phase 3 — The Pre-Maintenance Phase.
- Phase 4 is the Lifetime Maintenance Phase of the Atkins Diet program.

Read through the diet and make sure you understand it. If you are uncertain about something, Atkins has a very helpful team of people waiting to answer your questions. Reading through the diet will help you become more familiar with the foods you can eat on the different stages and what to avoid, especially in the Inductions Phase, which is the phase that trains your system to burn fat in your body.

Once you have familiarized yourself with the foods, check your pantry, refrigerator, and freezer to see what items you may already have. Make your grocery list and remember to note the carbs in your regular products. When you are at the grocery store, try to find similar low-carb alternatives.

CHAPTER 3: WORKING THROUGH PHASE 1 — THE INDUCTION PHASE OF THE ATKINS DIET

You will find the Atkins diet is easy to embrace and follow once you understand it. In this chapter, you are going to learn about each phase of the Atkins Diet. You will also become more familiar with the foods you can eat in each phase.

Phase 1 is the phase that most people who start the Atkins Diet plan start with. This is the phase where you cut down on your carbohydrate intake. Cutting down and controlling the number of carbohydrates you eat each day retrains the way your body burns fuel. Without the excess carbohydrates to store away, your body will start to burn fat.

Phase 1 is also the hardest part of the diet. I will not lie; the first few days I felt a little off my game. I am coffee-holic for one, so cutting down on my favorite beverage did not help my situation at all. I found drinking a lot of water, going for a walk around the garden, or even doing a few stretches helped. You can even try a bit of fresh mint/spearmint soaked in filtered water for a couple of hours or overnight. I found this helped me with any headaches and cravings and it filled me up.

No matter how hard it gets on Phase 1, the trick is not too quit. One of my favorite sayings is "When you are going through hell, keep going" (Winston Churchill). Push through the first week and the second week will not be that bad.

The Induction Phase of the Atkins diet usually lasts two weeks. You can stay on the Induction Phase for much longer should you need to. You can extend the two-week Induction phase if:

- You feel you have not lost enough weight.
- You are not yet 15 pounds from your goal weight.

Starting Phase 1 — Induction

You must stick to the recommended daily carbohydrates you consume. If you work within the following simple guideline for Phase 1, you will get the results you are hoping for.

- In Phase 1, you can eat 20 grams of **net carbohydrates** per day.

- You can eat less but should never go below 18 grams per day. Always check with a dietician, nutritionist, or health care professional first.

- If you feel you need a few more grams of carbs, try not to go over 22 grams per day. If you are eating 22 grams per day, slowly try to reduce the number of carbs to 20 grams after a week.

- Divide your 20 grams of carbohydrates into the following:
  - Acceptable salad or cooked vegetable — Eat 12-15 grams per day.

- Limit your protein intake to:
  - 115-175 grams per day for those who are short to medium in height or build.

- You need to keep yourself hydrated by drinking at least eight glasses of water per day. It is natural for your body to water weight on a diet. This can lead a person to feel dizzy, lightheaded, or lacking energy. Keeping yourself hydrated is the key to counteracting this.

- It is important to eat three square meals a day.

- Do not skip meals or snacks. If you are not hungry at mealtime, rather have a small snack or appetizer. Skipping a meal could make you overeat at the next one.

- You can also eat four to five small meals per day if you are used to eating more than three meals a day. Try eating three meals with a snack in between each meal.

- Try not to go without eating for longer than six hours at a time. You should try to eat something every three to four hours.

- Do not overeat. Eat until you feel full and no more. If you have eaten your meal or snack and still feel hungry, have a glass of water.

- Be aware of hidden sugars in some low-carb foods. Always read the nutritional labels.

- In Phase 1, fruit is not recommended; instead, all the nutrients you need are gained from the vegetables and other acceptable foods that are listed below.

- For the first two weeks of the Atkins Diet, seeds and nuts are not on the acceptable foods list and should be avoided.

- Chickpeas, legumes, kidney beans, and similar foods that are a mix of proteins and carbohydrates should be avoided.

- It is advisable to take a multivitamin to ensure you are getting all the nutrients your body needs. This is especially true during this phase of the diet when your body is adjusting to the change in your eating habits.

- You can enjoy fats on the Atkins diet as it is essential for helping the body to absorb various vitamins.

- Try and cut down on how much you eat during meal and snack times. If you still feel hungry after a meal, have a glass of water or a low-carb snack. Keep in mind that the snack will add to your carb intake for the day.

- Try to cut back on the amount of caffeine you drink per day. You need to become aware of what products contain caffeine as well.

- Be careful using or consuming too much artificial sugar substitutes. A lot of them are harmful, can have a laxative effect, and some even contain carbs (up to 1 g per packet).

What You Can Eat

The table below lists the food groups and recommended daily or weekly amounts. The recommendations below are to help you achieve optimum health. They are also designed to get your body to start using fat as its major fuel source.

Food Group	Description	Amount	Per Day/Week
Beverages	Be aware of hidden sugars in certain beverages.	64 ounces (8 glasses) of liquid	Day
Dairy	No dairy except for certain cheeses,	3 to 4 ounces	Day

	cream, or butter.		
Dressings	Salad dressings can contain quite a lot of carbs and sugars. Read the labels carefully. Limit dressings and opt to make your own low carb ones.	3 grams or lower	As required
Eggs	Eggs are an excellent source of nutrients. Try to eat at least 1 a day. Keep in mind that 1 large boiled egg can contain up to 0.6 grams of carbohydrates.	2 to 3 eggs	Day
Fats and Oils	Fats and oils generally have no to very little carbs. However, there is strict guidance on the recommended daily allowance. Always check if fats or oils are safe to cook with. Certain oils should not reach high temperatures.	2 to 4 tablespoons	Day
Fish	Fish is a good source of many nutrients, protein, and good fats. However, your body needs a variety of proteins so it is a good idea to eat a variety of different meats each week.	4 to 6 ounces	2 to 3 times a week
Garnishes	If you want to garnish a salad or dish, try using low to no carb garnishes.	1 large hard boil egg (0.6 g carbs) ½ cup sautéed mushrooms (1 g carbs)	As required
Herbs	Herbs are a great way to add flavor to a dish. When buying herbs, opt for fresh herbs. You can use dried herbs if you do check the label for any added sugar.	Up to 1 tablespoon	As required
Meat	Use only fresh meat and avoid	4 to 6 ounces	2 to 3 times a

	processed meats. This includes meat such as some bacon products, ham, and other processed cold meats. Be aware of any added nitrates that have been added to meat products.		week
Poultry	Poultry is another good source of protein. Although there are no carbs, like fish, you should only eat it a few times a week.	4 to 6 ounces	2 to 3 times a week
Shellfish	Shellfish is one of the best sources of essential nutrients such as zinc, iron, magnesium. It is also a source of Omega fatty acids, protein, and other healthy fats. You should keep in mind that some shellfish contain carbs.	Up to 4 ounces	2 to 3 times a week
Spices	Spices add flavor to any dish. Some spices like cayenne pepper can aid in weight loss. Always check for added sugar when choosing a spice brand. You can use salt but limit it and try to use only a pinch at a time.	Up to 1 tablespoon	As required
Sweeteners	Be wary of sweeteners. Some sweeteners are not good for your health. Opt for the more natural sweeteners like Stevia. One packet can also contain up to 1 g of carbs.	3 packets or teaspoons	Day
Vegetables	When you measure vegetables, you need to do so when they are raw. For the first two weeks. stick to the acceptable foods list for the foundation vegetables. Never drop below 12 g of these vegetables per serving if possible.	12 to 15 g	Day

Food List for Phase 1

The following is a list of the acceptable foods for each of the above categories. They contain a basic guide to the recommended portion size and total (net) carbs for each. This list is an excellent reference to help you choose your foods per meal and quickly put together a balanced meal.

Food	Amount	Net Carbs
Beverages		
Almond milk — unflavored and unsweetened	1 cup	1 g
Club soda	1 glass	0 g
Coffee — Decaffeinated or caffeinated (carbs measured for black coffee with no added sugar)	1 cup	0 g
Coconut milk — Unflavored and unsweetened	1 cup	2 g
Cream — Light	3.5 ounces	3.7 g
Diet soda (check the label for hidden sugars)	1 glass	0 g
Soy milk — Unflavored and unsweetened	1 cup	4g
Tea — Regular (carbs measured for black tea with no added sugar) Tea — Herbal (carbs measured for herbal tea with no added sugar)	1 cup	0 g
Water — Sparkling, still, mineral, tap, or spring	1 glass	0 g
Dairy		
Blue cheese	1 tablespoon	0.2 g
Cheddar cheese	1 ounce	0.4 g
Cream cheese	1 tablespoon	0.4 g
Feta cheese	1 ounce	1.2 g
Goat cheese	1 ounce	0.3 g

Gouda cheese	1 ounce	0.6 g
Mozzarella cheese	1 ounce	0.6 g
Parmesan cheese — Grated	1 tablespoon	0.2 g
Swiss cheese	1 ounce	1.0 g
Dressings		
Balsamic vinegar	1 tablespoon	2.7 g
Blue cheese salad dressing	1 tablespoon	2.3 g
Caesar salad dressing	1 tablespoon	1 g
Greek salad dressing	1 tablespoon	0.5 g
Italian salad dressing — Creamy	1 tablespoon	1.5 g
Lemon juice	1 tablespoon	1 g
Lime juice	1 tablespoon	1.2 g
Ranch salad dressing	1 tablespoon	0.7 g
Red wine vinegar White wine vinegar	1 tablespoon	0 g
Eggs		
Boiled	1 large egg	0.3 g
Devilled	1 large egg	2 g
Fried	1 large egg	0.6 g
Omelets	1 large egg	0.4 g
Poached	1 large egg	0.4 g
Scrambled	1 large egg	2 g
Fats and Oils		
Butter	1 tablespoon	0 g

Mayonnaise (with no added sugar)	1 tablespoon	0 g
Canola oil Coconut oil Grape seed oil Olive oil Safflower oil Sesame oil Soybean oil Sunflower oil Walnut oil	1 tablespoon	0 g
Fish		
Cod Flounder Halibut Herring Salmon Sardines Sole Trout Tuna	4 ounces	0 g
Garnishes		
Bacon — Crumbled (make sure there is no added sugar)	3 slices	0 g
Cream — Sour	tablespoon	0.6 g
Egg — Hard boiled	1 large egg	0.6 g
Cheese — Grated (different cheeses have different carb counts)	tablespoon	varies
Mushrooms — Sautéed	½ cup	1 g
Herbs		
Basil, Cilantro, Dill, Oregano, Tarragon	1 tablespoon	0 g
Chives	1 tablespoon	0.1 g
Garlic	1 clove	0.9 g

Ginger	1 tablespoon	0.8 g
Parsley	1 tablespoon	0.1 g
Rosemary	1 tablespoon	0.8 g
Sage	1 teaspoon	0.8 g
Meat		
Bacon	4 ounces	1.6 g
Beef	4 ounces	0 g
Ham	4 ounces	4.3 g
Lamb Pork Veal Venison	4 ounces	0 g
Poultry		
Chicken Cornish hen Duck Goose Turkey Ostrich	4 ounces	0 g
Shellfish		
Clams	4 ounces	0.7 g
Crab	4 ounces	0.5 g
Crayfish, Shrimp, Lobster	4 ounces	0 g
Mussels	4 ounces	3.4 g
Oysters	4 ounces	3.1 g
Squid	4 ounces	0.8 g

Spices		
Black pepper	1 teaspoon	0.9 g
Cayenne pepper	1 teaspoon	0 g
Salt — A dash/pinch of salt (0.4g) is 155 mg dietary sodium.	1 pinch	0 g
White pepper	1 teaspoon	0.9 g
Sweeteners — Choose a brand that has zero carbs if you can. 1 Packet = 1 tsp		
Saccharine Stevia Sucralose	1 packet	0 to 1 g
Vegetables		
Alfalfa sprouts — Raw	½ cup	0 g
Artichoke — Pickled/marinated	1	1 g
Arugula — Raw	½ cup	0.2 g
Asparagus — Cooked	6 stalks	1.9 g
Avocado — Raw	½	1.3 g
Beet greens — Cooked	½ cup	1.8 g
Bell pepper green — Raw	½ cup	2.2 g
Bell pepper red — Raw	½ cup	3 g
Bell pepper yellow — Raw	½ cup	3 g
Bok choy — Cooked	½ cup	0.4 g
Broccoli — Cooked	½ cup	1.8 g
Broccoli rabe — Cooked	½ cup	1.2 g
Broccolini — Cooked	3	1.9 g
Brussel sprouts — Cooked	½ cup	3.5 g

Button mushroom — Raw	½ cup	0.8 g
Cabbage — Cooked	½ cup	2.7 g
Cauliflower — Cooked	½ cup	1.7 g
Celery — Raw	1 stalk	1 g
Cherry tomato — Raw	10	4.6 g
Chicory greens — Raw	½ cup	0.1 g
Collard greens — Cooked	½ cup	1 g
Cucumber — Raw	½ cup	1.6 g
Dill pickles	1	1 g
Eggplant — Cooked	½ cup	2.3 g
Endive — Raw	½ cup	0.1 g
Escarole — Raw	½ cup	0.1 g
Fennel — Raw	½ cup	1.8 g
Garlic — Minced	2 tablespoons	5.3 g
Green beans — Cooked	½ cup	2.9 g
Kale — Cooked	½ cup	2.4 g
Kohlrabi — Cooked	½ cup	4.6 g
Leeks — Cooked	2 tablespoons	3.4 g
Lettuce — Raw	½ cup	0.5 g
Okra — Cooked	½ cup	1.8 g
Olives black — Raw	5	0.7 g
Olives green — Raw	5	0.1 g
Onion red/white — Raw	2 tablespoons	1.5 g
Portobello mushroom — Cooked	1	2.6 g

Pumpkin — Cooked	½ cup	4.7 g
Radish — Raw	1	0.2 g
Radish (daikon/white) — Raw (grated)	½ cup	1.4 g
Rhubarb — Raw	½ cup	1.8 g
Sauerkraut — Drained	½ cup	1.2 g
Scallion — Raw	½ cup	2.4 g
Shallot — Raw	2 tablespoons	3.4 g
Snow peas — Cooked	½ cup	5.4 g
Spaghetti squash — Cooked	½ cup	4 g
Spinach — Raw	½ cup	0.2 g
Sprouts/mung beans — Raw	½ cup	2.2 g
Swiss chard — Cooked	½ cup	1.8 g
Tomato small — Raw	1	2.5 g
Turnip greens — Cooked	½ cup	0.6 g
Turnip — Cooked	½ cup	2.4 g
Watercress — Raw	½ cup	0.1 g
Yellow squash — Cooked	½ cup	2.6 g
Zucchini — Cooked	½ cup	1.5 g

What Foods You Should Avoid

When you start with the Induction Phase of the Atkins Diet, there are foods you need to stay away from. The list below will give you a basic outline of which foods are not on the acceptable food and beverage list for Phase 1.

Foods to Avoid for Phase 1

Alcohol
During the Induction Phase, **no alcohol** is allowed. The consumption of alcohol may slow down your weight loss. In Phase 2, you can start to re-introduced a limited amount to your diet plan.
Baked Goods and Desserts
Stay away from all baked goods such as cakes, cookies, biscuits, muffins, pretzels, savory pies, bread, and rolls.
Avoid all kinds of desserts such as puddings, mousse, flan, pies, donuts, and so on.
Dairy
Flavored milk
Ice cream
Milk
Milkshakes
Yogurt drinks
Yogurt — Sweetened/flavored
Diet/Low-Fat Foods
You have to be very careful with foods marked both diet or low-fat.
Low-fat foods may still contain quite a bit of sugar.
Diet foods may still contain a high carb content.
Fruit
No fruit may be eaten during Phase 1.
Grains
Barely
Rice

Rye
Spelt
Wheat
Processed Foods
Processed food has gone through a process such as being ground, cured, rolled, etc.
Potato chips are an example of processed food, chopped ham, most bought baked goods, and so on.
Although some processed foods are not bad for you, you cannot eat them during Phase 1 of the Atkins Diet.
Some examples of **healthier processed** foods are:
Crackers made with whole-grains
Dried fruit
Ground corn tortillas
Frozen vegetables
Pasta made with whole-grains
Pitas made with whole-grains
Pizza bases made with whole-grains
Rice — brown
Rolled oats
Steel-cut oats
Refined Foods
Whole food is a food you can take straight from the garden and eat it. Whole food has a significantly higher nutrient value than its refined counterpart. Refined food is a food that has been picked/harvested and refined into another form. It will no longer contain the same nutrient value as did in its whole form.
Some examples of refined foods are:

Cakes
Cookies
Pasta — There are some pasta brands that are refined, especially white pasta.
Pastries
Potato chips
Pretzels
Rice — Some rice is refined, especially white rice.
Wheat bread
White flour
White sugar
Wraps
Starchy/High Carb Vegetables/Legumes
You cannot eat starchy vegetables during Phase 1 of the Atkins diet; some examples are starchy vegetables are:
Beans — Black, cannellini, kidney, navy, and pinto
Butternut squash
Carrots
Chickpeas
Corn
Lentils
Parsnips
Peas
Potatoes
Sweet potatoes

Turnips
Yams
Sweetened Beverages
Cordials
Ice coffees/teas
Fizzy flavored sodas
Slushies
Smoothies — high carb
Sweets
All sweets, including shaved ice, ice pops, lollipops, boiled sweets, toffies, chocolates, gummy sweets, mints, chewing gum, etc. should be avoided. If you have a sweet tooth, try a low-carb smoothie, health bar, or low-carb snack.

Meal Plan

Below is a seven-day example meal plan for Phase 1 of the Atkins Diet. When planning your meals:

- Do not exceed your daily net carb allowance.
- Counting you net carbs:
  - Net carbs = Total Carbohydrates - Fiber
  - If there is Sugar Alcohols listed, the calculation will be:
    - Net carbs = Total Carbohydrates - Fiber - Sugar Alcohols
- You can calculate your net carbs by using the "Net Carb Calculator," which you can download onto an Android or iOS mobile device. You can find the app in your mobile application store or go to the Atkins website: https://www.atkins.com/how-it-works/free-tools/mobile-app

- To discover the net carb count of as many foods as humanly possible - <u>You can download a handy carb counter in PDF format by clicking this link.</u>

- There are quite a few different carb counting apps available but it is advisable to get the one designed for the Atkins Diet.

- If you are at a loss, Atkins has their own brand of foods that are quick and easy to make. They offer Atkins Frozen Food and Meals, Atkins Bar, Atkins Shake, Atkins Treats, and more.

- The Atkins website provides useful information about where to buy their diet products from: <u>https://www.atkins.com/products</u>.

- Some large chain stores and Amazon also stock certain Atkins products. Always make sure you are buying true Atkins products when purchasing from the internet.

Phase 1 Seven-Day Meal Plan Example

Drink at least eight glasses of water a day to keep yourself hydrated.

Monday	
Breakfast	2 eggs, scrambled Served with: 2 oz smoked salmon ¼ tsp black pepper 1/2 avocado
Snack	1 Pepperoni stick
Lunch	A mixed green salad consisting of: 5 green olives 1.3 oz feta cheese 3 cherry tomatoes ½ tbsp white wine vinegar and 1 tbsp virgin olive oil dressing Topped with: 3 slices of crumbled bacon garnish
Snack	1 celery stalk stuffed with 2 tbsp of cream cheese

Dinner	3 oz tuna Mixed with: 1 tbsp mayonnaise 2 tbsp baby spinach, chopped 1 tbsp cheddar cheese — grated Baked for 8 to 10 minutes on: 2 portobello mushrooms
Tuesday	
Breakfast	2-egg omelet Filled with: 2 tbsp grated cheddar cheese 2 tbsp chopped spinach leaves 3 cherry tomatoes
Snack	Atkins snack bar — Peanut Butter Protein Wafer Crisps
Lunch	2 oz ground beef burger patty Cooked with: 1 oz grated cheddar cheese 1 tbsp white onions finely chopped Served on: ½ cup cauliflower — grated
Snack	1 grilled chicken leg
Dinner	2 poached eggs Served in: 1 Hass avocado (medium) — halved Topped with: 2 oz smoked salmon 1 tsp dill ¼ tsp black pepper
Wednesday	
Breakfast	2 boiled eggs Served with: 3 slices of cooked bacon 4 cherry tomatoes Fried in:

	2 tsp vegetable or coconut oil
Snack	1 oz string cheese
Lunch	2 0z lean beef strips Stir-fried with: 1 tbsp shallots — chopped ½ cup broccoli ½ cup eggplant — cubed
Snack	4 cherry tomatoes Topped with: 1 tbsp grated mozzarella ¼ tsp fresh basil dash of black pepper Grill for 5 to 8 minutes
Dinner	3 oz lean chicken breast Grilled with: ¼ tsp fresh crushed garlic ¼ cup of button mushrooms a dash of black pepper Served with: ½ cup cooked spaghetti squash
Thursday	
Breakfast	3 oz smoked salmon Served with: ¼ cup cucumber — chopped 1 tbsp cream cheese
Snack	½ avocado, Hass
Lunch	2 oz shrimp Served with: ¼ cup crisp lettuce leaves — shredded 2 green olives 2 black olives 1 tbsp cucumber — julienned 2 tsp mayonnaise
Snack	1 medium red bell pepper

	Stuffed with: 1 tbsp cream cheese Topped with: ¼ tsp dill a dash of black pepper
Dinner	2 oz trout Grilled with: 3 cherry tomatoes ¼ tsp crushed garlic dash of black pepper Served with: green leaf salad drizzle with a dressing made up of: 3 tsp olive oil 1 tsp white wine vinegar 1 tsp fresh chopped basil 1 packet of Stevia
Friday	
Breakfast	2 egg omelet Stuffed with: 1 tbsp vegetables of your choice from the approved vegetable list 1 tbsp grated cheddar cheese
Snack	Atkins Vanilla Latte Iced Coffee Protein Shake
Lunch	meatballs Served on: ½ cup mashed cauliflower
Snack	1 oz string cheese
Dinner	Pork chops — grilled ½ cup mixed vegetables from the approved vegetable list
Saturday	
Breakfast	½ avocado, Hass Topped with: 1 tbsp cream cheese

	dash of black pepper ½ tsp fresh basil — chopped 3 slices of lean bacon — diced
Snack	1 celery stalk Stuffed with: 1 tbsp cream cheese
Lunch	2 oz lean beef strips Sautéed with: a dash of black pepper ½ portobello mushroom — chopped 1 tbsp green bell pepper — chopped
Snack	Atkins snack bar - the low-carb pick of your choice
Dinner	Chicken salad, mix together: ¼ cup lettuce — shredded 4 green olives 1 tbsp feta cheese 1 tsp watercress 1 tbsp arugula (rocket) ¼ avocado — cubed 2 oz grilled white chicken meat — shredded Drizzle with: 1 tbsp olive oil 2 tsp red wine vinegar dash of cayenne pepper 1 tsp fresh crushed basil
Sunday	
Breakfast	2 boiled eggs Mashed with: 2 tbsp grilled/microwaved button mushrooms 3 cherry tomatoes A dash of black pepper
Snack	1 Pepperoni stick
Lunch	2 oz roast chicken ½ cup mixed vegetables from the approved vegetable list

Snack	Atkins Chocolate Banana Shake
Dinner	Leftover roast chicken kebabs ½ cup of mixed vegetables from the approved vegetable list

Adding to the Diet's Benefits with Exercises for Phase 1

The Atkins Diet is effective without exercise; however, it is encouraged, and if you can exercise, it can be beneficial to both weight loss and your health. There are many benefits to adding an exercise routine to your day, especially when you are on a diet.

Benefits of Exercise

The benefits of exercising are many-fold. Exercise helps:

- Your body burns fats.
- You achieve your weight loss goal.
- You maintain your optimal weight goal.
- You build muscle to tone your body.
- Maintain healthy joints, bones, and muscle tissue.
- Reduce the risk of developing diseases such as heart disease, diabetes, and high blood pressure.
- Reduce the risk of high cholesterol as it helps to maintain cholesterol levels in the body.
- With depression and anxiety.
- Control a person's stress levels.
- To have a positive effect on a person's psychological well-being.
- To improve a person's self-confidence. It can cut down on mood swings and make you feel more energetic and alert.

Establishing an Exercise Routine in Phase 1

If you have not exercised before or have not exercised for a while, you will need to ease into exercising. If you have any pre-existing conditions, you should check with your doctor first and consult with a trained physical fitness instructor. There are many benefits to exercising but, at the same time, you need to know your body's limitations.

Although focusing on getting your body into peak physical condition is something to work towards, you do not have to kill yourself to get there. For someone who is into sports or competes at a high level, their bodies are trained to be exercising machines. Most normal people may go for a hike, or take a walk, play a bit of tennis, or go for a jog. You are not looking to win any competitions or become a sports star.

There has been a lot of research over the last few decades that have shown even light exercise has benefits (Metcalfe, 2019). You don't have to become a cardio ninja to increase your body into a fitter state. If you want to become a fitness goddess, then you will need to focus on intense cardio workout mixed with weights, etc.

But, to start with, you can try a few of these exercises to build up your strength:

- To start, you should set your goal for 15 to 20 minutes a day, at least two to three times a week.
- Gradually increase this to 30 minutes a day and a few more days a week.
- Always do at least three to five minutes of stretching before you begin any type of exercise.
- Take a brisk 15 to 20-minute walk once or twice a day. Walking the dogs is good exercise.
- Taking a hike that has dips and inclines for 10 to 20 minutes. Be careful of the terrain you choose and always make sure you have someone with you.
- Do some gardening for 30 minutes; even raking, weeding, and digging are physical activities that can increase your fitness level.
- Do laps in a pool for 10 to 20 minutes as swimming is fun and excellent exercise.

- Cycling for 10 to 15 minutes is excellent for getting your heart rate to increase and working those muscles.

- Yoga or pilates is light, can be relaxing, and is an excellent way to relieve stress, anxiety, as it relaxes you.

Find a workout or type of exercise you enjoy. It does not have to be high impact as long as it gets you moving and your blood flowing. As mentioned above, a stroll around the garden twice a day to water your plants or do some planting also counts as exercise, as does raking the garden.

Playing and being active with the kids is another way to get some exercise in. Then there are exercises you can do while sitting down. These are low-impact callanetic type exercises. If you have stairs in your house, you take a walk up and down them a few times. Instead of taking your car to the market cycle or walk there, as long as it is safe to do so, that is. Every little helps and the more active you get, the more active you will want to become.

CHAPTER 4: WORKING THROUGH PHASE 2 — CONTINUED WEIGHT LOSS PHASE OF THE ATKINS DIET

Phase 2 is the phase that builds your daily allowed carb count up a bit. You can start to introduce some foods and beverages that you could not eat in Phase 1 into your daily diet.

The Continued Weight Loss Phase of the Atkins diet usually lasts one to two weeks. Phase 2 should last up until you are within 10 pounds of your goal weight.

Progressing to Phase 2 — Continued Weight Loss

As in Phase 1 of the Atkins Diet plan, in Phase 2, it is important that you stick to the recommended daily carbohydrate goal. Below are a few simple guidelines to help make the transition from Phase 1 to Phase 2 as simple as possible:

- In Phase 2, you can eat 25 grams of carbohydrates per day.

- You can eat less but should never go below 18 grams per day.

- Remember to check with a dietician, nutritionist, or health care professional first before starting any new diet regime. If you have any pre-existing conditions, even transitioning from one phase of the diet to the next should be carefully monitored.

- Try not to exceed your daily carb limit as your body should be used to 20 grams a day by this phase of the diet. If you feel hungry, try drinking a glass of water or eating a no/low-carb snack.

- Divide your 20 grams of carbohydrates into the following:
  - Acceptable salad or cooked vegetable — Eat 12-15 grams per day.
- Limit your protein intake to:
  - 115-175 grams per day for smaller framed builds.
  - 225 grams per day for men or women with a larger/taller frame build.
- Hydration is still key to keeping yourself from feeling hunger, dizzy, lightheaded, and maintaining good health.

- You still need to eat either three meals a day or four to five smaller ones.

- Have at least one to two low-carb or zero-carb snacks a day in between meals.

- Do not skip your meals even if you only have a snack at mealtime should you not feel hungry.

- Try to eat every three to four hours, once again even if it is just a light snack or low-carb to a zero-carb smoothie.

- Do not overeat during any meal or snack time; remember water fills you up nicely.

- In Phase 2, you can start to introduce various fruits back into your diet plan.

- In Phase 2, you can start to introduce a limited number of nuts and seeds back into your diet plan.

- In Phase 2, you can start to introduce moderate alcoholic drinks back into your diet plan.

- Keeping control of your portion size is highly recommended and will keep the pounds from coming back.

- The Atkins Diet does not recommend caffeine but still allows it in moderation.

- Try not to use a lot of salt, salt products, and artificial sweeteners.

What You Can Eat

The table below lists the food groups and recommended daily or weekly amounts for Phase 2 of the Atkins Diet. The food groups listed below are in addition to the food groups listed in Phase 1.

Food Group	Description	Amount	Per Day/Week
Alcohol	Limit alcohol. Use diet/carb-free drink mixes. Drink a glass of water before drinking alcohol as it can dehydrate you. Opt for spirits, red or white wines.	1 small glass	Day
Beverages	Always opt for water as your beverage of choice.	64 ounces (8 glasses) of	Day

		liquid	
Dairy	You can add a few more dairy items to the list of approved food for Phase 2.	Varies depending on the type of dairy	Day
Dressings	Salad dressings — same as in Phase 1	3 grams or lower	As required
Eggs	Eggs — same as in Phase 1	2 to 3 eggs	Day
Fats and Oils	Fats and oils — same as in Phase 1	2 to 4 tablespoons	Day
Fish	Fish — same as in Phase 1	4 to 6 ounces	2 to 3 times a week
Fruit	You can introduce certain fruits to your diet in Phase 2.	¼ cup	Day/week
Garnishes	Garnishes — same as in Phase 1	1 large hard boiled egg (0.6 g carbs) ½ cup sautéed mushrooms (1 g carbs)	As required
Herbs	Herbs — same as in Phase 1	Up to 1 tablespoon	As required
Juices	There are certain fruit juices that you can start adding to your diet in Phase 2.	2 tablespoons	As required
Legumes	Legumes can be added to your diet. These can be cooked or canned.	Varies depending on the type of legume	Day/week
Meat	Meat — same as in Phase 1	4 to 6 ounces	2 to 3 times a week
Nuts	Various nuts are allowed in Phase 2 of the diet.	Varies depending on	Week

		the type of nut	
Poultry	Poultry — same as in Phase 1	4 to 6 ounces	2 to 3 times a week
Seeds	There are certain seeds you can eat in Phase 2 of the diet.	Varies depending on the type of seed	Week
Shellfish	Shellfish — same as in Phase 1	Up to 4 ounces	2 to 3 times a week
Spices	Spices — same as in Phase 1	Up to 1 tablespoon	As required
Sweeteners	Sweeteners — same as in Phase 1	3 packets or teaspoons	Day
Vegetables	Vegetables — same as in Phase 1 Legumes can be eaten; please refer to Legumes below.	12 to 15 grams	Day

Food List for Phase 2

The following is a list of the acceptable foods for each of the above categories that you can enjoy in Phase 2 of the Atkins Diet. Please note that these foods are in addition to the food list laid out in Phase 1.

Food	Amount	Net Carbs
Alcohol		
Brandy Bourbon Gin Rum Scotch Whisky Vodka	1.5 fl. oz	0 g
Sherry — Dry	1.5 fl. oz	2 g
Red wine	6 fl. oz	2 g
White wine	6 fl. oz	1 g
Beverages		
All beverages in Phase 1 apply to Phase 2.		
Use diet beverages as mixes for alcohol	1 glass	0 g
Use diet tonic as a mix for alcohol	1 glass	varies
Dairy		
All dairy in Phase 1 apply to Phase 2.		
Cottage cheese (2%)	½ cup	4.1 g
Heavy cream	¾ cup	4.8 g
Ricotta cheese	½ cup	3.8 g

Yogurt — unsweetened, whole milk, Greek	½ cup	3.5 g
Yogurt — unsweetened, whole milk, plain	½ cup	5.5 g
Dressings, Eggs, Fats and Oils, and Fish		
All the above food groups listed in Phase 1 apply to Phase 2.		
Fruit		
Blackberries	¼ cup	1.6 g
Blueberries	¼ cup	4.5 g
Boysenberries	¼ cup	4.5 g
Cantaloupe	¼ cup	2.9 g
Coconut — unsweetened shredded/fresh	¼ cup	2.3 g
Cranberries	¼ cup	1.9 g
Gooseberries	¼ cup	3.9 g
Honeydew	¼ cup	3.5 g
Raspberries	¼ cup	1.7 g
Garnishes, Herbs, Meat, Poultry, Shellfish, Spices, Sweeteners, and Vegetables		
All the above food groups listed in Phase 1 apply to Phase 2.		
Juices		
Lemon juice	2 tablespoons	2 g
Lime juice	2 tablespoons	2.4 g
Tomato juice	4 ounces	4 g
Legumes		

Black beans	¼ cup	6.5 g
Chickpeas	¼ cup	10.9 g
Great northern beans	¼ cup	10.6 g
Kidney beans	¼ cup	5.9 g
Lima beans	¼ cup	6.1 g
Navy beans	¼ cup	10.1
Pinto beans	¼ cup	6.1 g
Nuts		
Almonds	24 nuts	2.2 g
Brazil nuts	6 nuts	1.4 g
Cashews	2 tablespoons	5.1 g
Macadamias	10 nuts	1.4 g
Peanuts	2 tablespoons	3.8 g
Pecans	2 tablespoons	3.8 g
Pine nuts	2 tablespoons	2 g
Pistachios	2 tablespoons	3 g
Walnuts	12 nuts	1.7 g
Seeds		
Pumpkin seeds	2 tablespoons	2 g
Sesame seeds	2 tablespoons	2 g
Sunflower seeds — hulled	2 tablespoons	1.5 g

What Foods You Should Avoid

In Phase 2, there are a few foods that you can start to introduce into your diet plan. However, there are still many foods you need to avoid; the table below lists the foods that you should avoid.

Foods to Avoid for Phase 2

Alcohol
As you read in the acceptable foods list above, during this phase you can start to enjoy certain alcoholic beverages in moderations. You should, however, avoid the following alcoholic beverages:
Alcoholic coffees
Alcoholic iced coffees
Alcoholic ice-creams
Alcoholic milkshakes
Ale — Both dark and light ale
Beer — Including light beers/ non-alcoholic beer
Brandy
Champagne
Cider
Cocktails
Cream-based liqueurs
Dessert wines
Liqueurs
Mocktails
Port

Sherry
Sparkling wines
Stout
Baked Goods and Desserts
You will still need to stay away from the baked goods listed in Phase 1.
With a higher carb intake, you can make low-carb desserts that fit within your daily carb allowance.
Dairy
You will still need to stay away from the dairy items listed in foods to avoid in Phase 1.
Diet/Low-Fat Foods
Always check for hidden sugars in any low-fat or diet food.
Fruit
Only eat the fruits on the approved food list for Phase 2.
Grains
You need to stay away from the grains as listed in foods to avoid in Phase 1.
Processed Foods
You need to stay away from all processed foods as listed in foods to avoid in Phase 1.
Refined Foods
You need to stay away from refined foods as listed in foods to avoid in Phase 1.
Starchy/High Carb Vegetables/Legumes
Only eat the higher carb vegetables and legumes that are listed in the approved food list for phase 2.
Sweetened Beverages
You must avoid any sweetened beverages as listed in Phase 1 foods to avoid list.

Sweets	
You still cannot eat any sweets and the same rules apply as listed in the sweets to avoid in Phase 1.	
For a sweet tooth, try one of the Atkins low-carb snack bars.	

Meal Plan

Below is a seven-day example meal plan for Phase 2 of the Atkins Diet. When planning your meals:

- Do not exceed your daily net carb allowance of 25 g per day.
- Try to vary your protein sources each day and week.
- Counting your net carbs:
  - Net carbs = Total Carbohydrates - Fiber
  - If there is Sugar Alcohols listed, the calculation will be:
    - Net carbs = Total Carbohydrates - Fiber - Sugar Alcohols
- You can download various apps from your mobile device's app store.
- You can download the Atkins Net Carb Calculator app from the Atkins website. (All the information is listed in the Meal Plan section of Phase 1.)

Phase 2 Seven-Day Meal Plan Example

Drink at least eight glasses of water a day. It is important for your optimum health to stay hydrated.

Monday	
Breakfast	Pumpkin, Almond, and Vanilla Whey Protein Sour Cream Pancakes (see Recipe 7)
Snack	6 Brazil nuts and 12 walnuts

Lunch	2 oz ground beef burger patty Topped with: ½ Hass avocado — sliced 1 slice tomato 1 slice cheddar cheese 2 tsp mayonnaise Serve between: 2 grilled portobello mushrooms
Snack	Atkins low-carb shake (no more than 4 g carbs)
Dinner	1.5 oz lamb steak — grilled Served with: 3 oz of cauliflower — mashed Mashed with: 2 tbsp cheddar cheese — grated 2 slices of fresh tomato A dash of ground black pepper 1 tsp mustard
Tuesday	
Breakfast	2 Atkins crisp bread Topped with: ½ Hass avocado — sliced 4 slices of cucumber 1 tbsp feta cheese — crumbled a dash of black pepper drizzled with lemon juice
Snack	2 oz Greek yogurt 1 tbsp blueberries
Lunch	2 oz salmon fillet — grilled 2 tbsp feta cheese — crumbled 1 tbsp cashew nuts Served on: ¼ baby spinach leaves a dash of ground black pepper
Snack	¼ honeydew melon

Dinner	2 oz roasted chicken Served with: ¼ cup pumpkin — cooked ¼ cup Brussels sprouts — cooked 1 portobello mushroom — grilled ¼ tsp crushed garlic a dash of cayenne pepper
Wednesday	
Breakfast	Chocolate, Mint, and Avocado Smoothie (see Recipe 32)
Snack	Atkins snack (no more than 4 g net carbs)
Lunch	Salad made with: ¼ baby spinach leaves 2 tbsp feta cheese 1 tbsp raspberries 1 tbsp blueberries 1 tsp pine nuts Salad dressing made from: 1 tbsp white wine vinegar 1 tsp olive oil 1 tsp fresh basil 2 packets of Stevia
Snack	¼ cup strawberries
Dinner	Vegetable Lamb Stew (see Recipe 19)
Thursday	
Breakfast	2-egg omelet Filled with: 1 oz smoked salmon ½ tsp capers 1 tsp dill ¼ tsp cayenne pepper 2 tbsp feta cheese — crumbled
Snack	¼ cup strawberries
Lunch	2 oz grilled chicken — shredded

	Mixed into the following salad: ¼ cup brown mushrooms — sautéed ¼ cup baby spinach leaves — shredded ¼ cup iceberg lettuce leaves — shredded 2 tbsp blue cheese — crumbled (replace with feta if desired) 1 tsp roasted sesame seeds Topped with the following dressing: 1 tsp olive oil 3 tsp red wine vinegar a dash of ground black pepper
Snack	Atkins Iced Coffee Milkshake
Dinner	Chicken kebabs made from: 3 oz grilled white chicken meat — cubed ¼ cup red bell pepper — sliced ¼ cup shallots — sliced ¼ cup brown mushrooms — halved Place chicken and vegetables onto kebab sticks and grill. Serve on a bed of: ¼ cup baby spinach — slightly cooked
Friday	
Breakfast	2 eggs — scrambled Scrambled with: 1 tbsp scallions — chopped 1 tbsp fresh baby spinach — shredded 1 tbsp cheddar cheese — shredded 1 tbsp feta cheese — crumbled
Snack	1 Atkins crisp bread Topped with: 1 tbsp chunky cottage cheese 3 green pitted olives — halved a dash of cayenne pepper
Lunch	Artichoke and Sesame Seed Salad (see Recipe 9)
Snack	12 walnuts and 1 tsp sesame seeds
Dinner	Beef Stroganoff on a Bed of Green Bean (see Recipe 15)

Saturday	
Breakfast	Berry Coconut Breakfast Parfait (see Recipe 5)
Snack	1 tbsp honeydew melon and 1 tbsp cranberries or raspberries
Lunch	Hearty Cream of Asparagus Soup (see Recipe 12)
Snack	Atkins snack (no more than 4 g net carbs)
Dinner	Filet Medallions with Blackberry, Feta, and Spinach Salad (see Recipe 16)
Sunday	
Breakfast	Breakfast Blueberry Muffins (see Recipe 3)
Snack	Atkins shake — a flavor of your choice (no more than 4 g net carbs)
Lunch	Portobello Beef Burger with Feta and Spring Onion (see Recipe 14)
Snack	1 tbsp pumpkin seeds
Dinner	Lamb Chops with Cauliflower Mash (see Recipe 17)

Adding to the Diet's Benefits with Exercises for Phase 2

If you have been exercising through Phase 1, you should, by now, be ready to slightly increase your routine. That is if you are physically able to and there are not any issues that prevent you from doing so.

You may want to try to include the following few exercises into your routine:

- Stretch

Start with a three to five-minute stretch. You can either lie on the floor on a mat. Lift your arms over your head and stretch your legs out. Point your toes to feel the stretch in your calves.

Bring your arms down and lift one knee to your chest. Hold for five seconds and repeat the stretch with your other knee.

Roll up into a sitting position with your legs folded in front of you. Roll your neck to one side, then pivot it around the back to the other side and roll it around the front.

Take two deep breaths and stretch your arms up above your head, then out in front of you, before rolling into a standing position.

Take a deep breath and stretch your arms up as if you can lift yourself up on your toes as you stretch. Breathe out and relax the stretch; repeat one more time.

Lift your foot up to your buttocks, hold for a few seconds, release and repeat with the other leg. If you cannot balance, make sure to hold onto a firm structure for support.

Remember to stretch after you have exercised as well.

- Arm rolls

To firm up your arms, hold your arms out to the sides with your fingers up. Rotate your arms around in small circles 20 times backward and 20 times forward. You can gradually increase these as you feel you can do more.

- Squats

Hold on to the back of a chair if you are unable to balance. Make sure your feet are planted firmly on the floor and facing forward but slightly apart. Keep your back straight, head up, then squat. Sink into the squat like you are about to sit on a chair. Do 5 to 10 repetitions and gradually increase these as your strength improves.

- Crunches

Standing crunches are just as good as the ones you do lying down. Stand with your buttocks squeezed tight and shoulders back. Suck your tummy in. Put your arms out in front of you. As you pull your arms back towards your body, ball your hands into fists as if you are pulling a weight. Tilt your pelvis forward, make sure to suck in your tummy. You should feel the stretch in your belly. Hold for two seconds, release, and repeat for 20 to 30 crunches.

For lying down crunches, position a mat on the floor. Lie down flat on the mat. Pull your knees up and suck your belly in picturing your belly button pulling towards your spine. Place your hands behind your head and tilt your chin towards your chest.

Do NOT pull your crunch up with your arms as this only strains your neck. You need to feel the crunch by using your stomach muscles to lift your upper body. Do not swing into a full sit-up either. You need to gently lift your upper body until your shoulders are not on the floor. Keep your buttocks tight, tummy sucked in, and your lower back on the floor. Hold the crunch of a second before releasing it.

Do 5 to 10 of these and gradually increase the number of crunches as you feel stronger. Remember, if you can feel the crunch in your neck, you are pulling up wrong. Your head and neck should remain relaxed while you are crunching.

- Push-Ups

You are probably thinking *"Agh, I hate those"*; well these are push-ups with a difference. To increase your arm strength, you can lean against a sturdy counter or even a wall. It is best to start off with the wall.

Stand with your palms flat against the wall and an arm's length away from the wall. Your feet should be shoulder-width apart and facing forward. Keep your shoulders straight, chin up, and buttocks and stomach must be pulled tight. Allowing your full weight to lean in towards the wall. It is like doing a push-up standing up. Make sure to bend your elbows as you lean forward, pull them in against your body.

Push away from the wall, straightening your elbows as you stand back up straight. Do not remove your hands from the wall. Repeat the process for 10 to 15 repetitions, which you can increase as your strength does.

For a harder version of this push-up: lean at a slight angle against a countertop. But make sure your feet are flat on the floor.

Well done! You have worked hard to get through the second phase of the Atkins diet. Keep going you are closing in on your goals.

CHAPTER 5: PHASE 3 — PRE-MAINTENANCE PHASE OF THE ATKINS DIET

If you have advanced to Phase 3, congratulations as you should only have approximately 10 pounds to lose to reach your goal weight.

Continuing on to Phase 3 — Pre-Maintenance

Phase 3 is called the Pre-Maintenance Phase as it is designed to get you to your goal weight, and then help you maintain that weight for at least four weeks. This means that this phase can last from six to eight weeks, depending on how rapidly you drop those last few extra pounds.

- In Phase 3, you can eat 30 grams of carbohydrates per day until you have lost your desired weight.

- Once you have reached your goal weight, you need to maintain that weight for at least four weeks thereafter.

- During those four weeks, you need to slightly increase your carbohydrate intake by 5 to 10 grams a day each week.

- By the time you are ready to progress to Phase 4, you should be eating approximately 80 to 100 grams of carbohydrates a day. This amount depends on how your body responds to the higher carb rate. If you feel you are putting on weight, drop the amount down by 5 grams.

- As you introduce more starchy foods into your body, you will be able to figure out how your body responds to them. If you feel bloated or uncomfortable, you know to leave that food out altogether. Watch your carb count closely when introducing higher carb foods.

- Before you start a new phase of the Atkins Diet, always check with a dietician, nutritionist, or health care professional. This will ensure you can apply to continue with the plan or if you need to adjust the diet.

- Try not to go over your set daily allowed carbohydrate consumption.

- Your daily amount of carbohydrates should include 12 to 15 grams of acceptable foods and vegetables.
- Limit your protein intake to 115-175 grams per day.
- Drink at least eight glasses of water per day.
- Eating three square meals a day is a must and you should not skip meals or snacks.
- Eat four to five smaller meals a day rather than three if you find this helps stave off hunger and stops any cravings.
- Try and eat something every three to four hours. Never go longer than six hours without eating.
- Always be on the lookout for hidden sugars in all foods and beverages.
- Keep your portion size down to the amount that leaves you feeling full. You don't want to feel like you are stuffed or bloated after a meal.
- Don't overeat; eat until you're full.
- Keep alcohol and caffeine to a minimum.

What You Can Eat

The food groups for Phase 3 remain the same as they were in Phase 2. However, there are a few foods that can be reintroduced into your diet plan in this Phase.

Acceptable Food List for Phase 3

The following is a list of the acceptable foods that you can enjoy in Phase 3 of the Atkins Diet. Please note that these foods are in addition to the food lists laid out in Phase 1 and Phase 2.

Food	Amount	Net Carbs
Alcohol		
All acceptable alcohol in Phase 2 applies to Phase 3.		
Beverages, Dairy, Dressings, Eggs, Fats and Oils, Fish, Garnishes, Herbs, Juices, Legumes,		

Meat, Poultry, Shellfish, Spices, Sweeteners, and Vegetables.		
All the above food groups listed in Phase 1 and Phase 2 apply to Phase 3.		
Fruit		
All fruit in Phase 1 and 2 apply to Phase 3.		
Apple	½ fruit	7.9 g
Apricot — medium	3 fruit	9.6 g
Banana — small	1 fruit	20.4 g
Cherries	¼ cup	5.3 g
Clementine	1 fruit	7.6 g
Coconut — fresh and unsweetened shredded	½ cup	2.5 g
Dates — fresh	3 fruit	15.8 g
Figs — fresh	1 fruit	4.5 g
Grapes — red	½ cup	13 g
Grapefruit — medium	½ fruit	8.9 g
Guava	½ cup	7.4 g
Kiwi	1 fruit	8.1 g
Mango	½ cup	11.1 g
Orange	½ cup	14.5 g
Papaya	½ cup	6.6 g
Peach — small	1 fruit	10.5 g

Pineapple	½ cup	9.7 g
Plum — medium	1 fruit	6.6 g
Pomegranate seeds	¼ cup	6.4 g
Watermelon	½ cup	5.5 g
Grains — amounts can vary depending on the brand		
Barley — cooked	½ cup	19.2 g
Bread — whole wheat	2 slices	20 g
Grits — cooked	½ cup	15.2 g
Millet — cooked	½ cup	19.5 g
Oat bran	2 tablespoons	6.0 g
Oatmeal	⅓ cup	19 g
Pasta — whole wheat and cooked	½ cup	16.6 g
Polenta	2 tablespoons	12.5 g
Quinoa — cooked	¼ cup	8.6 g
Rice — brown and cooked	½ cup	21.2 g
Wheat bran	2 tablespoons	1.6 g
Wheat germ	2 tablespoons	4.9 g

Nuts		
All nuts in Phase 1 and 2 apply to Phase 3.		
Pine Nuts	2 tablespoons	0.8 g
Poultry		
All poultry in Phase 1 and 2 apply to Phase 3.		
Seeds		
All seeds in Phase 1 and 2 apply to Phase 3.		
Poppy seeds	1 tablespoon	1.2 g
Pumpkin seeds	2 tablespoons	2.4 g
Sesame seeds	2 tablespoons	2.1 g
Vegetables — Starchy		
Acorn squash	½ cup	7.6 g
Beets	½ cup	6.8 g
Butternut squash	½ cup	8.5 g
Carrots	½ cup	4 g
Corn	½ cup	14.9 g
Parsnips	½ cup	10.2 g

Peas	½ cup	7 g
Potato — baked, medium	½ potato	13.1 g
Sweet potato — baked, medium	½ potato	9.9 g
Rutabaga	½ cup	5.9 g

What Foods You Should Avoid

Phase 3 is a little more lenient with the foods you may eat as long as you watch your crabs and remain within your daily allowance. You should still stay away from the obvious foods such as sugary sweets, drinks, and starchy foods or hidden sugars loaded with carbs.

Cutting back on alcohol is still advised, and sticking to the approved list alcohol choices still apply. Remember to only use low-carb or zero soda choices as alcohol mixers and to include a few glasses of water in between alcoholic drinks to avoid dehydration.

Exercise

In Phase 3, you should have a little more energy and your body will be used to the reduced carbohydrate intake. You can increase your exercise routine to what you are comfortable with and fits into your busy schedule. If you find you have to squeeze exercise into your lifestyle, it will start to feel like a chore and you may just give it up altogether.

If you are comfortable with your current routine, up your reps a bit and add 5 to 10 minutes more onto your workout time.

Reaching Your Goal Weight

Upon reaching your goal weight, you will continue on Phase 3 for another four weeks. You will gradually need to increase your carbs by 5 grams at a time. You will need to increase your carb intake amount during these 4 weeks until you reach around 80 grams per day.

Staying on Phase 4 for another four weeks helps you get used to eating at a normal daily carb intake and get used to doing so. You will need to keep a careful eye on your meals, the food you eat, and your weight. Having done this for the past six or more weeks, this should not be that hard.

Carry on making your low-carb meals with some added carbs to pad your intake to your new amount. You can start to add some low-carb baked goods or even increase your snack size. Just remember to keep within your limits and don't fall back into your bad eating habits.

CHAPTER 6: PHASE 4 — LIFESTYLE MAINTENANCE PHASE OF THE ATKINS DIET

Reaching Phase 4 is a huge milestone for you. It means you have reached your goal weight and managed to keep it constant for the past four weeks. Well done!

Phase 4 is the Continuous Maintenance Phase and goes on indefinitely. It is the phase where you transition from the Atkins Diet to the Atkins Lifestyle.

Food List for Phase 4

The following is a list of the acceptable foods that you can enjoy in Phase 4 of the Atkins Diet. Please note that these foods are in addition to the food list laid out in Phase 1, Phase 2, and Phase 3.

Food	Amount	Net Carbs
Alcohol,		
All acceptable alcohol in Phase 2 and 3 apply to Phase 4.		
Beverages, Dairy, Dressings, Eggs, Fats and oils, Fish, Garnishes, Grains, Herbs, Juices, Legumes, Meat, Nuts, Poultry, Seeds, Shellfish, Spices, Sweeteners, Starchy Vegetables, and Vegetables		
All acceptable food groups listed in Phase 1, 2, and 3 apply to phase 4.		
Fruit		
All fruit in Phase 2, and 3 apply to Phase 4.		
Pear — medium	1 fruit	21 g
Raisins	1 tablespoon	6.8 g
All legumes in Phase 1 and 2 apply to Phase .4.		

Staying in Control

Phase 4 is all about sticking to your new low-carb eating plan. If you have done so up until now, it should be easy to continue making low-carb food choices. The list of approved foods is not a definitive one; there are loads of low-carb food choices out there. By this phase, you should be on at least 80 grams to 100 grams of carbs per day.

You just need to check the foods you are buying to ensure that they fit into your healthy eating regime. If you do eat high-carb food at a meal or for a snack, make sure you adjust the daily limit around it. There are a lot of low- to no-carb foods that can fill you up for your next meal or snack.

The more adventurous you are with your recipes and food experimentation, the wider your low-carb food choice will become. Try new foods, beverages, and baked goods or treats. In the modern-day, there are a lot of substitutes for the sugary treats and the beverages you love. For instance, use sugar-free low-carb cool drink syrup to make tasty fizzy drinks with club soda or sparkling water. Choose sugar-free maple or caramel syrups to bake with and sugar replacements such as Stevia.

Don't think about the ending of a diet or even keep the word diet, eating plan, or lifestyle in your head. Rather just move with your new flow and keep refining your eating habits as you live your life the low-carb way.

CHAPTER 7: ATKINS FOR VEGANS AND VEGETARIANS

With people opting for plant-based lifestyles, there are now a lot of food substitutes for meat, fish, poultry, and dairy products on the market that are suitable for vegans and vegetarians. The Atkins diet has come a long way since it was first developed and can now be adapted to suit vegan, vegetarian, and pescatarian eating plans.

Some studies have shown that eating a plant-based diet is beneficial to a person's health. Even women who are not vegetarians or vegans will benefit from eating plant-based diets every now and again. They offer nutrient dense meals that do not put a strain on the metabolism as much as consuming meat does.

Health benefits of a plant-based diet include:

- Lowers high blood pressure
- Improve gut function
- Lower cholesterol
- Boost the immunes system
- Reduce inflammation

Vegan

The Atkins Diet can be adjusted to suit the eating preference of vegans. Phase 1 of the Atkins Diet has a lot of restrictions on foods such as nuts, legumes, berries, fruit, and some vegetables. As a vegan, you may find it difficult to start the diet on Phase 1 as you do not eat eggs or dairy products. It is, therefore, recommended that those who follow meat- and dairy-free eating lifestyles start at Phase 2 of the Atkins 20 Diet Plan.

Adapting the Atkins Diet Plan for Vegans

Make the following adjustments to adapt the Atkins diet to a vegan lifestyle:

Start the diet in Phase 2 - Ongoing Weight Loss Phase (OWL)

- Start with 50 g of net carbs per day to lose weight.

- Each week, increase your daily net carb intake by five grams.

- NOTE: Only increase carbs each week if you are losing weight. If not, do not increase your carb limit until you have lost at least one to two pounds.

- Stay in Phase 2 for two weeks.

- You can stay in Phase 2 for up to four weeks if you have not come within 10 lbs of your goal weight.

- When you are 10 lbs from your goal weight, progress to Phase 3 — Pre-Maintenance Phase.

- If you want to maintain your weight and only have 10 lbs or less to lose, start the diet in Phase 3.

- Start Phase 3 with 60 grams of net carbs per day.

- In Phase 3, you can increase your net carbs by five grams per week until you reach 80 grams per day, but only increase your carbs if you are losing weight.

- When you have achieved your goal weight, you will stay on Phase 3 without increasing your carb count for another four weeks. This is to make sure you are maintaining your weight at that carb intake level per day.

- If you have maintained your weight for four weeks, you will move into Phase 4, which is the Maintenance and Lifestyle Phase of the diet.

- In Phase 4, you will continue to eat as you did in Phase 3 but you will be able to experiment with more food types as long as you stick to the recommended daily carb intake.

- The meal plans in Phase 2 in Chapter 4 can be adapted to suit a vegan eating plan.

- The Atkins 100 Diet plan is a great plan for vegans to follow.

- Vegans should take a flax oil supplement.

Foods

The following is a list of foods that are acceptable on the Atkins Diet for vegans; the list is similar to that of Phase 1 and Phase 2 as laid out in the chapters above. For your convenience, I have converged the two lists, taken out the non-vegan foods. I have added some substitute foods for protein and fat replacements. For any beverages that are not listed below, see the lists in the non-vegan Phase 1 to Phase 3 lists in the chapters above.

Food	Amount	Net Carbs
Phase 2 - Ongoing Weight Loss		
Beverages		
Coffee — Decaffeinated or caffeinated (carbs measured for black coffee with no added sugar)	1 cup	0 g
Tea — Regular (carbs measured for black tea with no added sugar) Tea — Herbal (carbs measured for herbal tea with no added sugar)	1 cup	0 g
Water — Sparkling, still, mineral, tap, or spring	1 glass	0 g
Dairy Substitutes		
Almond milk — unsweetened, organic	¼ cup	2 g
Coconut cream	1 tablespoon	3.1 g
Coconut milk — unsweetened, organic	¼ cup	3 g
Soya milk	¼ cup	3.5 g
Dressings		
Balsamic vinegar	1 tablespoon	2.7 g
Lemon juice	1 tablespoon	1 g
Lime juice	1 tablespoon	1.2 g
Red wine vinegar	1 tablespoon	0 g

White wine vinegar		
Egg Substitute		
Silken tofu — scrambled egg substitute, organic	1 oz	2 g
Vegg — scrambled egg substitute, Vegg — egg yolk substitute	¼ cup	0 g
Vegan Egg	1 large egg	0.6 g
Fats and Oils		
Almond butter	¼ cup	0.4 g
Canola oil, Grape seed oil, Olive oil, Sesame oil, Soybean oil, Sunflower oil, Walnut oil	1 tablespoon	0 g
Coconut butter	1 tablespoon	0.8 g
Macadamia butter	1 tablespoon	0.4 g
Fruit		
Blackberries	¼ cup	1.6 g
Blueberries	¼ cup	4.5 g
Boysenberries	¼ cup	4.5 g
Cantaloupe	¼ cup	2.9 g
Coconut — unsweetened shredded/fresh	¼ cup	2.3 g
Cranberries	¼ cup	1.9 g
Gooseberries	¼ cup	3.9 g
Honeydew	¼ cup	3.5 g
Raspberries	¼ cup	1.7 g

Herbs		
Basil, Cilantro, Dill, Oregano, Tarragon	1 tablespoon	0 g
Chives	1 tablespoon	0.1 g
Garlic	1 clove	0.9 g
Ginger	1 tablespoon	0.8 g
Parsley	1 tablespoon	0.1 g
Rosemary	1 tablespoon	0.8 g
Sage	1 teaspoon	0.8 g
Juices		
Lemon juice	2 tablespoons	2 g
Lime juice	2 tablespoons	2.4 g
Tomato juice	4 ounces	4 g
Legumes		
Black beans	¼ cup	6.5 g
Chickpeas	¼ cup	10.9 g
Great northern beans	¼ cup	10.6 g
Kidney beans	¼ cup	5.9 g
Lima beans	¼ cup	6.1 g
Navy beans	¼ cup	10.1
Pinto beans	¼ cup	6.1 g

Meat Substitutes		
Coconut meat	1 ounce	1.7 g
Eggplant	3 ounces	2 g
Portobello mushrooms — medium	2 mushrooms	4 g
Quorn — cutlets	3 ounces	3.7 g
Seitan	3 ounces	0.2 g
Soybeans	¼ cup	0.2 g
Tofu	3 ounces	0.5 g
Nuts		
Almonds	24 nuts	2.2 g
Brazil nuts	6 nuts	1.4 g
Cashews	2 tablespoons	5.1 g
Macadamias	10 nuts	1.4 g
Peanuts	2 tablespoons	3.8 g
Pecans	2 tablespoons	3.8 g
Pine nuts	2 tablespoons	2 g
Pistachios	2 tablespoons	3 g
Walnuts	12 nuts	1.7 g
Seeds		

Chia seeds	2 tablespoons	2 g
Flaxseeds	2 tablespoons	0.2 g
Hemp seeds	2 tablespoons	0.5 g
Poppy seeds	2 tablespoons	2.4 g
Pumpkin seeds	2 tablespoons	2 g
Sesame seeds	2 tablespoons	2 g
Sunflower seeds — hulled	2 tablespoons	1.5 g
Spices		
Black pepper	1 teaspoon	0.9 g
Cayenne pepper	1 teaspoon	0 g
Salt — A dash/pinch of salt (0.4 g) is 155 mg dietary sodium.	1 pinch	0 g
White pepper	1 teaspoon	0.9 g
Sweeteners — Choose a brand that has zero carbs if you can. 1 Packet = 1 tsp		
Saccharine Stevia Sucralose	1 packet	0 to 1 g
Vegetables		
Alfalfa sprouts — Raw	½ cup	0 g
Artichoke — Pickled/marinated	1	1 g
Arugula — Raw	½ cup	0.2 g

Asparagus — Cooked	6 stalks	1.9 g
Avocado — Raw	½	1.3 g
Beet greens — Cooked	½ cup	1.8 g
Bell pepper green — Raw	½ cup	2.2 g
Bell pepper red — Raw	½ cup	3 g
Bell pepper yellow — Raw	½ cup	3 g
Bok choy — Cooked	½ cup	0.4 g
Broccoli — Cooked	½ cup	1.8 g
Broccoli rabe — Cooked	½ cup	1.2 g
Broccolini — Cooked	3	1.9 g
Brussel sprouts — Cooked	½ cup	3.5 g
Button mushroom — Raw	½ cup	0.8 g
Cabbage — Cooked	½ cup	2.7 g
Cauliflower — Cooked	½ cup	1.7 g
Celery — Raw	1 stalk	1 g
Cherry tomato — Raw	10	4.6 g
Chicory greens — Raw	½ cup	0.1 g
Collard greens — Cooked	½ cup	1 g
Cucumber — Raw	½ cup	1.6 g
Dill pickles	1	1 g
Eggplant — Cooked	½ cup	2.3 g
Endive — Raw	½ cup	0.1 g
Escarole — Raw	½ cup	0.1 g
Fennel — Raw	½ cup	1.8 g

Garlic — Minced	2 tablespoons	5.3 g
Green beans — Cooked	½ cup	2.9 g
Kale — Cooked	½ cup	2.4 g
Kohlrabi — Cooked	½ cup	4.6 g
Leeks — Cooked	2 tablespoons	3.4 g
Lettuce — Raw	½ cup	0.5 g
Okra — Cooked	½ cup	1.8 g
Olives black — Raw	5	0.7 g
Olives green — Raw	5	0.1 g
Onion red/white — Raw	2 tablespoons	1.5 g
Portobello mushroom — Cooked	1	2.6 g
Pumpkin — Cooked	½ cup	4.7 g
Radish — Raw	1	0.2 g
Radish (daikon/white) — Raw (grated)	½ cup	1.4 g
Rhubarb — Raw	½ cup	1.8 g
Sauerkraut — Drained	½ cup	1.2 g
Scallion — Raw	½ cup	2.4 g
Shallot — Raw	2 tablespoons	3.4 g
Snow peas — Cooked	½ cup	5.4 g
Spaghetti squash — Cooked	½ cup	4 g
Spinach — Raw	½ cup	0.2 g
Sprouts/mung beans — Raw	½ cup	2.2 g

Swiss chard — Cooked	½ cup	1.8 g
Tomato small — Raw	1	2.5 g
Turnip greens — Cooked	½ cup	0.6 g
Turnip — Cooked	½ cup	2.4 g
Watercress — Raw	½ cup	0.1 g
Yellow squash — Cooked	½ cup	2.6 g
Zucchini — Cooked	½ cup	1.5 g

Phase 4 Foods

In Phase 4 of the Atkins diet, vegans may start to re-introduce some starchy vegetables along with some whole grain foods.

The foods listed below are to be added to the list above.

Fruit		
All fruit in Phase 1 and 2 apply to Phase 3.		
Apple	½ fruit	7.9 g
Apricot — medium	3 fruit	9.6 g
Banana — small	1 fruit	20.4 g
Cherries	¼ cup	5.3 g
Clementine	1 fruit	7.6 g
Coconut — fresh and unsweetened shredded	½ cup	2.5 g
Dates — fresh	3 fruit	15.8 g

Figs — fresh	1 fruit	4.5 g
Grapes — red	½ cup	13 g
Grapefruit — medium	½ fruit	8.9 g
Guava	½ cup	7.4 g
Kiwi	1 fruit	8.1 g
Mango	½ cup	11.1 g
Orange	½ cup	14.5 g
Papaya	½ cup	6.6 g
Peach — small	1 fruit	10.5 g
Pineapple	½ cup	9.7 g
Plum — medium	1 fruit	6.6 g
Pomegranate seeds	¼ cup	6.4 g
Watermelon	½ cup	5.5 g

Grains		
Barley — cooked	½ cup	19.2 g
Bread — whole wheat	2 slices	20 g
Grits — cooked	½ cup	15.2 g
Millet — cooked	½ cup	19.5 g
Oat bran	2	6.0 g

		tablespoons	
Oatmeal		⅓ cup	19 g
Pasta — whole wheat and cooked		½ cup	16.6 g
Polenta		2 tablespoons	12.5 g
Quinoa — cooked		¼ cup	8.6 g
Rice — brown and cooked		½ cup	21.2 g
Wheat bran		2 tablespoons	1.6 g
Wheat germ		2 tablespoons	4.9 g

Vegetables — Starchy			
Acorn squash		½ cup	7.6 g
Beets		½ cup	6.8 g
Butternut squash		½ cup	8.5 g
Carrots		½ cup	4 g
Corn		½ cup	14.9 g
Parsnips		½ cup	10.2 g
Peas		½ cup	7 g
Potato — baked, medium		½ potato	13.1 g
Sweet potato — baked, medium		½ potato	9.9 g

Rutabaga	½ cup	5.9 g

Foods to Avoid

Avoid all refined foods, foods with sugar, and starchy vegetables that are not on the acceptable food list. For a more comprehensive list, you can see the foods to avoid in the chapter above for Phase 1.

Vegetarian

Vegetarians can benefit from the Atkins Diet. As per the vegan section above, due to not eating animal proteins, it is advisable for vegetarians to start at Phase 2 of the diet. As pasta and other refined foods are not recommended, excluding these from your diet will help you lose weight.

As you are substituting plant-based proteins for animal proteins, you have to be careful which ones you choose and keep track of the net carbs in them. If you eat eggs, this is a good source to stack your daily protein with.

Adapting the Atkins Diet Plan for Vegetarians

Make the following adjustments to adapt the Atkins diet to a vegetarian lifestyle:

Start the Diet in Phase 2 - Ongoing Weight Loss Phase (OWL)

- Start with 25 to 30 g of net carbs per day to lose weight.
- If you are steadily losing weight, you can increase your net carbs by five grams a day each week.
- Stay in Phase 2 for two weeks or up to four weeks if you have not come within 10 lbs of your goal weight.
- Phase 3 will start when you only have 10 more pounds to lose to reach your goal weight.
- Start Phase 3 with 40 grams of net carbs per day.

- In Phase 3, you can increase your net carbs by five grams per week until you reach 80 grams per day. If you are not losing weight steadily, do not increase your carbs.

- You will stay in Phase 3 until you have reached your goal weight.

- After you have achieved your goal weight, you will stay in Phase 3 for another four weeks to encourage you to keep your new eating habits. This phase is the phase that gets you ready to move onto the lifestyle phase.

- Once you have maintained your goal weight for up to four weeks, you will move onto Phase 4 the Maintenance or Lifestyle Phase.

- The meal plans in Phase 2 in the chapters above can be adapted to suit a vegetarian or pescatarian eating plan.

- As a vegetarian, it is highly recommended that you take either a fish oil or flax oil supplement to ensure you are getting enough nutrients in your diet.

Foods

You can follow the above vegan acceptable food list, which has a comprehensive list of meat substitutes, vegetables, legumes, fruits, nuts, etc. The list covers acceptable low-carb foods for Phase 2 and Phase 3. Phase 4 is the same as Phase 3, only you will now have the tools and knowledge to experiment with a wider variety of low-carb foods.

For acceptable beverages, including alcohol and dairy products, see the acceptable foods lists for Phase 1, Phase 2, and Phase 3 in the chapters above. You can adjust your food plan by following the tips below:

- If you eat fish and seafood (pescatarian), make sure you use a good portion of these to top up your protein. To get a rich source of Omega-3 fatty acids, try fish such as sardines, salmon, and mackerel.

- Eggs are a good source of protein and can be eaten scrambled, boiled, fried, or in an omelet form.

- Use vegetables such as scallions and herbs to add flavor to your dishes.

- Beans, such as kidney beans, navy beans, lima beans, and soybean are a good source of protein. They are also high in dietary fiber.

- Try meat replacement using vegetables like eggplant. When eggplant is sliced and fried or grilled, it makes a great substitute for bacon. You can use it as a garnish over salads, etc.

- Coconut meat is another good meat replacement and can also be used as a bacon substitute.

- Portobello mushrooms make a tasty replacement for steak. They are a versatile food that is rich in protein and other vital nutrients. You can grill them and use them to add a unique flavor to any salad or dish.

- Replace cow's milk, butter, and creams with nut butter and creams.

- Dairy milk is not allowed on most phases of the Atkins diet and substitutes, such as soy milk, almond, macadamia, and coconut milk, are recommended.

- Make sure you are getting enough fats in your diet.

- Avoid the starchy vegetables that are not on the approved list and eat lots of the vegetables that are on the approved list.

- Eat nuts and seeds to top up on superfoods along with berries and fruit.

- Be careful when eating fruit as there are quite a few carbs in most fruit.

Foods to Avoid

See the chapters above that cover foods to avoid for Phase 1 and Phase 2 as these are the foods that you should stay away from. They are mainly all refined foods, some high-carb starchy vegetables, and baked goods with lots of refined ingredients including sugar. Sweets, soda, and fast foods need to be avoided.

CHAPTER 8: LIVING THE ATKINS LIFESTYLE

By this chapter, you will have realized that living the Atkins lifestyle is not that difficult. Making healthier choices and watching your carb intake gets easier the more your practice. By the time you have gone onto the Maintenance Phase of the diet, you will already have started to retrain yourself to reach for the lower carb items. Even counting your carbs will soon become second nature to you.

In this chapter, we are going to look at keeping your spirits up, finding your motivation, dealing with slip-ups, and common mistakes to avoid. There are also some general tips for living the Atkins lifestyle and motivational stories.

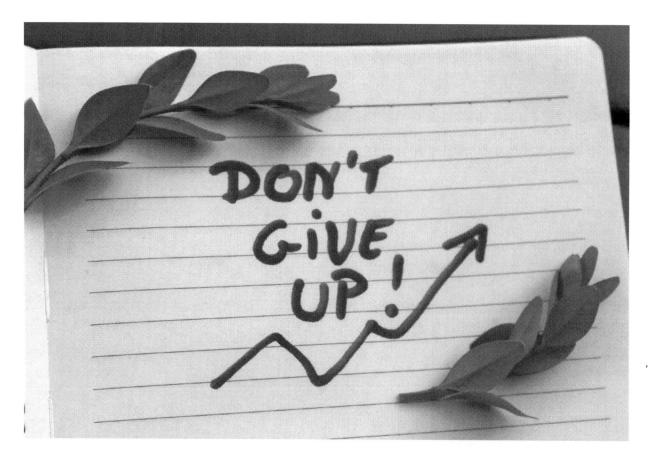

The Challenges Ahead

During your diet, you are going to run into many challenges ahead, most of which will come from yourself.

Slip-Ups and Temptations

It is very easy to get disheartened when dieting. No matter how hard you try, there are going to be times when you slip up or give in to temptation. It is natural and everyone does it. The important thing is how you deal with that slip-up.

Don't get disheartened or stressed out about slipping in and giving into temptation. There is no need to punish yourself. If you know you are going to do it again, rather pick a treat day and work your allocated daily carb limit around that day. This gives you a day to look forward to and will motivate you to stick to achieving your weekly goal.

The important thing is to know what your weaknesses are and how to overcome them. When it comes to dieting, most people's weakness comes from those very tempting sugary carb-filled treats and starchy comfort foods.

The trick to getting around your cravings for these foods is to find something that you can substitute for them. Then train yourself to think about those foods as your comfort treats. For example, if you love ice cream, use a low-carb sweet substitute and make yourself ice blocks. When you crave ice cream, crush the ice blocks in a cup to enjoy instead.

As you progress through the phases in the Atkins diet, you will be able to eat more foods. There are a lot of really tasty baked goods and treats you can make for yourself. Making your own treats is also a lot healthier than buying them from the store. You get to control what goes into the food.

If you find yourself wanting a cake or something sweet while at the store, buy a diet soda to sip on or a bottle of fizzy water. Try not to go to the store when you are hungry. This will increase your cravings for fast foods and treats. Before you go, fill yourself up with a few glasses of water and a low-carb snack. That way the tantalizing smell of the baked goods section won't be as tempting.

Try to keep your slip-ups to a minimum and avoid situations or places you know trigger them.

Some Common Mistakes to Avoid

When you first start out on the diet or even when you are a seasoned Atkins dieter, you can still make mistakes. Here is a list of common mistakes people tend to make on the Atkins Diet:

- Becoming obsessed with weighing or measuring yourself

You should weigh and measure yourself once a week. Make a set day to do this. Only weight or measure yourself on a different day if you miss your designated one. If you become obsessed with weighing yourself every day, you will start to either lose motivation or revert to starving yourself or over-exercising. Keep calm and trust in the process. As long as you are eating according to plan, you will lose those pounds.

- Not eating enough vegetables

You need to at least eat one or two vegetables on the acceptable food list a day. You need to make sure you are eating at least 15 grams of them a day.

- Not eating enough protein

Your body needs protein and you should be eating at least four ounces a meal. Be careful not to eat too much protein as this could interfere with your weight loss.

- Trying to avoid fats

Lots of people shy away from fats because they have a bad reputation in the nutritional world. There are indeed fats that are bad for you and should be avoided but there are also good ones that are essential for your health. The essential ones are the ones you need to help your body burn fat.

- Not taking notice of the carbs in foods

One of the major pitfalls when it comes to counting carbs is not reading labels or being aware of the hidden sugar in certain foods. Even foods that say they are low-carb or diet foods may have hidden sugars adding to higher carbs. There are many nutritional counter apps that you can quickly look upon if you are in doubt.

- Not counting carbs correctly

Another very common mistake is not counting the net carbs in food. You have to remember to subtract the dietary fiber from the total carbs on a nutrition label.

- Not keeping a journal

Keeping track of the diet is a way to stay motivated, keep yourself on the correct diet path, and take note of things like your progress and foods you like. It is also a great way to help you get in touch with how you feel about yourself. When you start, you may feel you have no confidence, etc. Journaling is a good source of motivation to see how your feelings progress along with your new eating plans

Keeping Motivated

Here are some tips on how to keep yourself motivated to move forward and stay on track:

- Remind yourself that you are doing this for you. To make you feel about yourself and your lifestyle.
- Don't look at yourself and see the weight that is not there.
- Keep yourself positive by being excited about finding out how much you lost each week.
- Even if you have managed to retain last week's weight loss, that is still a win. Congratulate yourself.
- If you, for some reason, gain a pound or two, don't fret. Try harder next week.

- Don't compare yourself to others. You are you, a unique individual with a body that may have the same sort of shape as another person but it is not the same. There are a lot of factors that make you different from another person.

- Be proud of who you are and what you are accomplishing.

- Don't let negative thoughts creep in. If they do, write them in your journal and tell them you will get back to them. Then write positive thoughts down on the next page that you are addressing today.

- Think of your new lifestyle as a great adventure and have fun with it.

The Atkins Lifestyle and Your Family

When you are on a diet and have a family, it can sometimes mean having to cook two separate meals. Having to cook two separate meals and watch your family eat the foods you enjoy while you eat steamed can quickly make you lose interest in a diet.

By the time you get to this section of the book, you will have seen that the foods you eat on the Atkins diet can be eaten by the entire family. You do, however, have to adjust the serving sizes to ensure your family members are getting enough carbohydrates and nutrients.

Always check with a health care provider, nutritionist, or dietician for your family's exact daily nutrition requirement, especially if they have any pre-existing conditions. The sections below give you an idea of what the recommended daily nutrition intake should be.

Adults

The recommended daily nutritional guideline for an average person consuming 2,000 calories per day:

- 200 g carbohydrates
- 25 to 30 g fiber
- No more than 50 g sugars
- 150 g protein

- No more than 70 g fat

- Less than 20 g saturated fat

- 300 mg cholesterol

- Less than 2,300 mg sodium

Healthy Food Plate for Adults

Picture a dinner plate with a glass on the side.

- Glass
    - At least 8 glasses of water
    - Dairy 1 to 2 servings per
    - Juice 1 small glass
- Plate
    - Moderate oils such as vegetable oils and fats, and keep trans fats to a minimum.
    - ½ of the plate should contain vegetables and fruits. Stay away or limit starchy vegetables like potatoes, etc.
    - ¼ of the plate should contain whole grains. For example, whole wheat, quinoa, brown pasta, brown rice, steel-cut oats, etc. Limit or cut out refined foods.
    - ¼ of the plate should be protein. For example, meat, fish, poultry, or meat substitutes.

Children

The recommended daily nutritional guideline for children changes with their age:

Daily Recommended Nutrition Guideline for Children 1 to 18							
Age	Sex	Calories	Carbs	Fiber	*Sugar	Protein	*Sodium
1 to 3	B & G	1,000 to 1,200	130 g	19 g	25 g	13 g	1,500 mg
4 to 8	G	1,200 to 1,800	130 g	25 g	25 g	19 g	1,900 mg

4 to 8	B	1,200 to 2,000	130 g	25 g	25 g	19 g	1,900 mg
9 to 13	G	1,400 to 2,200	130 g	26 g	25 g	34 g	2,200 mg
9 to 13	B	1,600 to 2,600	130 g	31 g	25 g	34 g	2,200 mg
14 to 18	G	1,800 to 2,400	130 g	29 g	25 g	46 g	2,300 mg
14 to 18	B	2,000 to 3,200	130 g	38 g	25 g	52 g	2,300 mg

*This is the maximum recommended daily allowance. Try to consume less if possible.

Healthy Food Plate for Children

Kids need the same healthy eating food plate breakdown as adults; this includes the fats and oil and beverages.

The table below is a guideline to recommended portions of food groups for kids:

Daily Recommended Nutrition Guideline for Children 1 to 18 based on the recommended calories in the table above.						
Age	Sex	Dairy	Fruits	Grains	Protein	Vegies
1 to 3	B & G	2 cups	1-1.5 cups	3-5 oz	2-4 oz	1-1.5 cups
4 to 8	G	2.5 cups	1-1.5 cups	4-6 oz	3-5 oz	1.5-2.5 cups
4 to 8	B	2.5 cups	1-2 cups	4-6 oz	3-5.5 oz	1.5-2.5 cups
9 to 13	G	3 cups	1.5-2 cups	5-7 oz	4-6 oz	1.5-3 cups
9 to 13	B	3 cups	1.5-2 cups	5-9 oz	5-6.5 oz	2-3.5 cups
14 to 18	G	3 cups	1.5-2 cups	6-8 oz	5-6.5 oz	2.5-3 cups
14 to 18	B	3 cups	2-2.5 cups	6-10 oz	5-5.7 oz	2.5-4 cups

CHAPTER 9: LOW-CARB BREAKFAST RECIPES

Here are seven easy-to-make low-carb breakfast recipes.

Please note that the nutritional information is per serving and that the carbohydrates reflect the **net carbs** and **not** the total carbs.

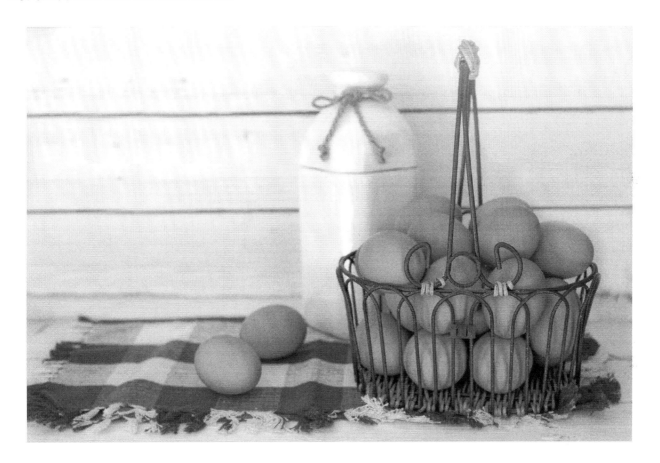

Recipe 1 — Quick and Easy Ham, Mozzarella Cheese, and Mushroom Omelette

This omelet is quick and easy to make. You can microwave the toppings for 1 minute before adding them to the omelet to ensure the ingredients are cooked.

You can add a few more carbs to the recipe by adding to an ingredient or adding another ingredient for diet Phases 3 and 4.

The recipe is suitable for Phase 1 to Phase 4.

Serving Size: 1

Time: 20 minutes

Prep Time: 10 minutes

Cook Time: 10 minutes

Nutritional Facts/Info:

- Calories 311
- Net Carbs 3.4 g
- Fiber 0.5 g
- Sugars 0.9 g
- Fat 21.9 g
- Protein 25.5 g

Ingredients:

- 2 large eggs
- 1 tbsp chopped ham
- 1 tbsp mozzarella cheese — shredded
- 1 tbsp brown mushrooms — chopped
- dash of black pepper
- 1 tsp coconut oil

Directions:

1. In a mixing bowl, beat eggs with a dash of black pepper.

2. Heat coconut oil in an omelet pan.

3. Pour the egg mixture into the pan.

4. Allow to cook for 1 minute, or until the omelet is cooked through.

5. Flip with a spatula and add the chopped ham, chopped mushrooms, and shredded cheese.

6. Flavor with a dash of black pepper.

7. Flip the one half of the omelet to cover the ingredients.

8. Flip the folded omelet and cook for 30 seconds to 1 minute.

9. Flip the folded omelet onto the other side for another 30 seconds.

10. Remove the pan from the heat and dish the omelet onto a breakfast plate.

Recipe 2 — Green Bell Pepper Stuffed With Steak and Baby Spinach

Bell peppers are a good source of iron. They make a delicious breakfast for a great start to the day.

If you are using this recipe for Phase 2 and up, you can add cream or cottage cheese to it to increase the net carbs.

The recipe is suitable for Phase 1 to Phase 4.

Serving Size: 1

Time: 25 minutes

Prep Time: 10 minutes

Cook Time: 15 minutes

Nutritional Facts/Info:

- Calories 162
- Net Carbs 3.9 g
- Fiber 2.2 g
- Sugars 3 g
- Fat 7.2 g
- Protein 18.7 g

Ingredients:

- 1.7 oz steak — cut into strips
- 1 medium green bell pepper — whole
- 1 tbsp brown mushrooms — diced
- 2 tbsp baby spinach leaves — shredded
- ¼ tsp garlic — crushed
- 1 tsp coconut oil or vegetable oil
- dash of black pepper

Directions:

1. In a skillet, heat the coconut or vegetable oil over medium heat.
2. Cook the steak to your cooking preference.
3. Add the crushed garlic, mushrooms, and spinach; sauté for 1 to 2 minutes. Add these ingredients 1 to 2 minutes before the steak is cooked.
4. Remove the ingredients from the pan and put on a plate to cool slightly.
5. Cut the top off the bell pepper and remove the seeds.
6. Using the same skillet you cooked the steak in, heat the green pepper to slightly soften it. Do not overcook it or burn it.
7. Remove the bell pepper from the skillet and place it on a plate.
8. Stuff the pepper with the steak mixture and serve.

Recipe 3 — Breakfast Blueberry Muffins

These muffins are cooked in the microwave and take only 15 minutes to make. They are great for an on-the-go breakfast.

The recipe is Suitable for Phase 2 to Phase 4.

Serving Size: 1

Time: 12 minutes

Prep Time: 10 minutes

Cook Time: 2 minutes

Nutritional Facts/Info:

- Calories 217
- Net Carbs 7.3 g
- Fiber 0.9 g
- Sugars 4.2g
- Fat 13.3 g
- Protein 15.8 g

Ingredients:

- 1 egg — at room temperature
- 3 tbsp blueberries — fresh or unsweetened if frozen
- ¼ tsp sesame seeds
- 2 tbsp whey protein powder — vanilla
- 2 tbsp cream cheese
- dash of nutmeg
- ¼ tsp baking powder
- ¼ tsp vanilla extract

Directions:

1. Whisk together the cream cheese and egg in a mixing bowl.

2. Add the baking powder, nutmeg, egg, vanilla extract, and whey protein powder.

3. Whisk together until the mixture is well mixed.

4. Mix in the sesame seeds and blueberries.

5. Pour the mixture into a microwavable mug.

6. Place the mixture in the mug into the microwave for 1 minute.

7. After a minute, test to see if the muffin is done by gently inserting a clean knife or skewers into the middle of it.

8. If the knife or skewer comes out clean, the muffin is done. If not, heat it for another 10 to 15 seconds at a time until the knife comes out clean when inserted into the middle.

9. Tip the muffin onto a cooling rack or plate to cool for a few seconds before eating it.

Recipe 4 — Smoked Salmon, Dill, and Avocado With Poached Egg

In phase 1, you can only use ½ the avocado, but as you progress to the next phase, you can use both halves of the avocado to increase the carb count. Avocados are a great source of good fats, high in fiber, and good for controlling cholesterol.

The recipe is Suitable for Phase 1 to Phase 4.

Serving Size: 1

Time: 15 minutes

Prep Time: 10 minutes

Cook Time: 5 minutes

Nutritional Facts/Info:

- Calories 310
- Net Carbs 3.5 g
- Fiber 7.3 g
- Sugars 0.9 g
- Fat 26.1 g
- Protein 12 g

Ingredients:

- 1 large egg
- 1 tbsp smoked salmon — shredded
- ½ avocado
- 3 cherry tomatoes — halved
- 1 tsp mozzarella cheese — shredded
- ¼ tsp dill
- dash of chili pepper (optional)
- dash of ground black pepper

Directions:

1. Poach the egg.
2. Place the halved cherry tomatoes in the halved avocado.
3. Place ½ the dill, ½ the mozzarella, and ½ the smoked salmon on top of the tomatoes.
4. Place the poached egg on top of the halved avocado.
5. Add the leftover dill, smoked salmon, and mozzarella on top of the poached egg.
6. Sprinkle a dash of chili pepper and freshly ground black pepper to taste.

Recipe 5 — Berry Coconut Breakfast Parfait

This parfait makes a great sweet and tangy breakfast meal. You can add a dash of cayenne pepper to give it some spice. If you feel you need a bit more sweetness, you can add another tsp of sweetener.

The recipe is Suitable for Phase 2 to Phase 4.

Serving Size: 1

Time: 15 minutes

Prep Time: 15 minutes

Cook Time: N/A

Nutritional Facts/Info:

- Calories 204
- Net Carbs 6.9 g
- Fiber 3.4 g
- Sugars 4.9 g
- Fat 16 g
- Protein 6.6 g

Ingredients:

- 1 tbsp blackberries — fresh, unsweetened if frozen
- 1 tbsp raspberries — fresh, unsweetened if frozen
- 2 medium strawberries — halved
- ¼ cup fresh coconut meat — shredded, unsweetened if bought shredded
- ¼ cup cream — heavy
- ¼ cup Greek yogurt — fat-free
- 2 tsp Stevia (2 x 1 g sachets) — you can use any of the acceptable sweeteners
- ½ tsp vanilla extract

Directions:

1. In a large mixing bowl, blend the yogurt, cream, vanilla, and 1 tsp of Stevia.

2. Blend the mixture with a whisk or blender on medium until mixture forms soft peaks.

3. Cut the blackberries and raspberries into halves.

4. Place ½ of the cut blackberries and ½ of the cut raspberries into a small mixing bowl.

5. Purée the berries in the small mixing bowl.

6. Fold the remaining blackberries and raspberries into the purée.

7. Gently mix 1 tsp (1 sachet) of Stevia into the pure mixture.

8. If you are using fresh coconut meat, chop it into bite-sized chunks.

9. In a parfait glass or breakfast bowl:

   o Scoop in 1 tbsp yogurt/cream mixture.

   o Top the yogurt with a sprinkling of coconut.

   o Top the yogurt with 1 tbsp berry purée mixture.

   o Top the berry purée with a sprinkling of coconut.

   o Continue layering the parfait until both mixtures are finished

   o The parfait works well if you end it with the yogurt mixture.

   o Leave enough coconut to sprinkle on the top of the parfait.

10. Top the parfait with the 2 halved fresh strawberries.

Recipe 6 — Goat Cheese, Asparagus, and Turkey Scramble

You can add 1 tbsp chopped tomato or ½ tsp roasted sesame seeds to this recipe from Phase 2 to Phase 4.

The recipe is Suitable for Phase 1 to Phase 4.

Serving Size: 1

Time: 25 minutes

Prep Time: 10 minutes

Cook Time: 15 minutes

Nutritional Facts/Info:

- Calories 273
- Net Carbs 1.9 g
- Fiber 1.2 g
- Sugars 1.9 g
- Fat 17.7 g
- Protein 25.5 g

Ingredients:

- 2 eggs
- 3 medium asparagus spears
- 1 oz turkey — shredded
- 1 oz goat cheese
- 1 tsp basil — shredded
- 1 tsp coconut or vegetable oil
- dash of black or red pepper to tastes

Directions:

1. In a mixing bowl, beat the eggs.

2. Add a dash of black pepper.

3. Chop the asparagus spears in bite-sized chunks.

4. Heat the oil in a skillet over medium heat.

5. Add the beaten eggs and stir in the asparagus.

6. When the eggs are done, remove them from the heat.

7. Add the turkey, goat cheese, and basil.

8. Add a dash of black pepper to taste and serve.

Recipe 7 — Pumpkin, Almond, and Vanilla Whey Protein Sour Cream Pancakes

You can enjoy these delicious pumpkin pancakes with a dollop of sour cream.

The nutritional information is calculated per pancake.

The recipe is Suitable for Phase 2 to Phase 4.

Serving Size: 6 pancakes

Time: 20 minutes

Prep Time: 10 minutes

Cook Time: 10 minutes

Nutritional Facts/Info:

- Calories 221
- Net Carbs 3.9 g
- Fiber 1.6 g
- Sugars 1.8 g
- Fat 12.4 g
- Protein 21.9 g

Ingredients:

- 4 large eggs — at room temperature
- ½ cup almond flour — blanched
- 1 tsp baking powder
- 4 oz whey protein — vanilla
- ½ cup cooked pumpkin — mashed
- ¼ low-fat plain cottage cheese — chunky
- ½ tsp pumpkin spice
- 3 tbsp sour cream
- 1 tbsp coconut or vegetable oil

Directions:

1. Beat the eggs in a mixing bowl.
2. In another mixing bowl, mix almond flour, cooked pumpkin, baking powder, and cottage cheese.
3. Whisk the beaten eggs into the almond flour mixture until the mixture is light and fluffy.
4. Add the pumpkin spice and stir it into the mixture well.
5. Lightly grease a large non-stick pan with coconut or vegetable oil. You can use butter to grease the pan as it will not add to the carbohydrate count. It does slightly increase the fat and protein count.
6. Heat the greased non-stick pan over a hot plate.
7. Each pancake takes approximately 3 tablespoons (¼ cup) of the mixture.
8. Using either a cup or tablespoon, scoop the mixture onto the heated non-stick pan.
9. You should be able to get at least 3 pancakes in a large pan at a time.
10. Turn the pancakes after about 2 minutes or when the pancake is firm.
11. Once the second side is done, remove the pancake from the heat.
12. Light grease and heat the pan once again.
13. Repeat steps 7 to 11 until you have used all the pancake batter.
14. Serve pancakes with a dollop (1 tsp) of whipped sour cream.

CHAPTER 10: LOW-CARB LUNCH RECIPES

Here are seven easy-to-make low-carb lunch recipes.

Please note that the nutritional information is per serving and that the carbohydrates reflect the **net carbs** and **not** the total carbs.

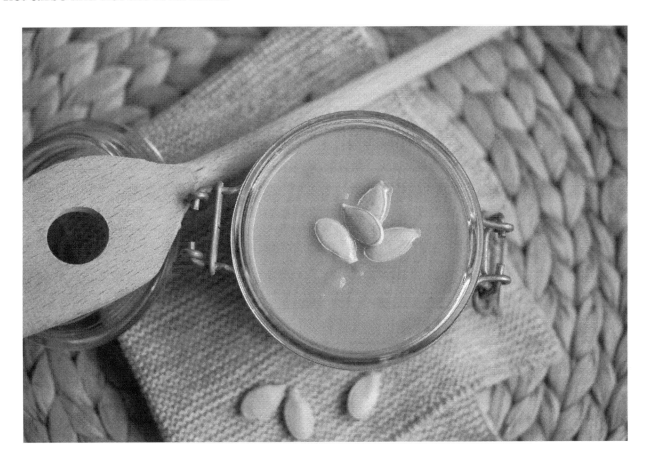

Recipe 8 — Portobello Mushrooms Topped With Red Bell Pepper, Zucchini, and Swiss Cheese

You can leave off the cheese for a dairy-free meal choice in phase 1. In phase 2, you can add ½ tbsp crushed cashews, which will add 1.3 g of net carbs to the recipe.

The recipe is suitable for Phase 1 to Phase 4.

Serving Size: 1

Time: 20 minutes

Prep Time: 10 minutes

Cook Time: 10 minutes

Nutritional Facts/Info:

- Calories 158
- Net Carbs 3.3 g
- Fiber 0.3 g
- Sugars 1 g
- Fat 11.7 g
- Protein 8.8 g

Ingredients:

- 1 large portobello mushroom
- 1 tbsp green bell pepper — finely chopped
- 1 tbsp zucchini — finely chopped
- 1 slice of Swiss cheese
- ¼ tsp butter
- ¼ tsp garlic — crushed
- cayenne pepper to taste

Directions:

1. Use ½ tsp butter to spread on the underside of the mushroom.

2. Spread the crushed garlic over the butter.

3. Heat the grill and place the portobello mushroom on the grill.

4. Grill for 3 to 5 minutes; the mushroom should be slightly tender.

5. Heat the chopped zucchini and green pepper with the leftover butter in the microwave for 1 minute.

6. Add a dash of cayenne pepper to the mix and stir it in well.

7. Place the heated zucchini and green pepper on the portobello mushroom.

8. Break the Swiss cheese and layer it over the zucchini and green pepper.

9. Place the portobello mushroom in the grill until the cheese has melted.

10. Remove from the grill when the cheese is slightly browned and it will be ready to serve.

11. If you are adding crushed cashews, add the cashews before you serve the mushroom.

Recipe 9 — Artichoke and Sesame Seed Salad

Try something different with this artichoke salad sprinkled with sesame seeds, pine nuts, watercress, and goat cheese.

The recipe is suitable for Phase 2 to Phase 4.

Serving Size: 1

Time: 10 minutes

Prep Time: 10 minutes

Cook Time: N/A

Nutritional Facts/Info:

- Calories 132
- Net Carbs 2.1 g
- Fiber 2 g
- Sugars 4.1 g
- Fat 12.3 g
- Protein 2.8 g

Ingredients:

- ½ Artichoke heart — marinated
- 2 tbsp cup watercress — chopped
- 1 tsp fresh basil — chopped
- 1 tsp roasted sesame seeds
- 1 tsp pine nuts
- 1 tbsp goat cheese — crumbled
- 1 tsp balsamic vinegar
- 1 tsp virgin olive oil
- 1 tbsp red wine vinegar
- 1 tsp Stevia or sweetener on the approved foods list

Directions:

1. Chop artichoke hearts into bite-sized pieces and place them in a medium-sized salad bowl.
2. Add chopped watercress, basil, sesame seeds, and pine nuts.
3. Crumble the goat cheese over the salad.
4. In a jar, mix the virgin olive oil, balsamic vinegar, red wine vinegar, and Stevia.
5. Shake the olive mixture well and drizzle over the artichoke salad.

Recipe 10 — Steak, Spinach, Avocado, and Brown Mushroom Bowl

This is a nice meal to eat either hot or cold. If you are going to eat it cold, you will only have to cook the steak. Use baby spinach leaves instead of regular spinach and do not cook the mushrooms.

To use it as a meal for Phase 2 and up, you can add some nuts, seeds, and cheese of your choice. Feta, goat cheese, or blue cheese complements this dish nicely.

You can leave off the mayonnaise and garlic sauce.

The recipe is suitable for Phase 1 to Phase 4.

Serving Size: 1

Time: 25 minutes

Prep Time: 10 minutes

Cook Time: 15 minutes

Nutritional Facts/Info:

- Calories 296
- Net Carbs 7.3 g
- Fiber 1.3 g
- Sugars 2.8 g
- Fat 19.4 g
- Protein 22.3 g

Ingredients:

- 2 oz steak — cut into strips
- ¼ spinach
- ¼ cup brown mushrooms — halved

- ½ avocado — Hass

- ¼ tsp garlic — crushed

- ¼ tsp mustard powder

- 1 tbsp mayonnaise

- black to taste

- dash of cayenne pepper

- 2 tsp coconut oil or vegetable oil

Directions:

1. In a small mixing bowl, mix together the mayonnaise, mustard powder, garlic, and a dash of cayenne pepper.

2. Cover the mayonnaise mixture and put it into the refrigerator.

3. Heat coconut or vegetable oil in a large skillet.

4. Add the steak strips and sear for 1 to 2 minutes.

5. Add the mushroom and allow to cook with the steak for 1 to 2 minutes.

6. Rip the spinach into large shreds and add to the skillet.

7. Flavor with black pepper to taste.

8. Remove when the steak is cooked to your liking.

9. The spinach and the mushrooms should be soft and not overcooked.

10. Add the steak mixture into a bowl.

11. Drizzle with the mayonnaise mixture.

12. Slice the avocado half into strips and add it to the top of the steak mixture.

Recipe 11 — Salmon, Avocado, and Feta Green Leaf Salad

Salmon and feta cheese make a mouthwatering combination when paired in a salad.

If you are using this salad in Phase 2 to Phase 4, add 1 tbsp blackberries and some pine nuts.

The recipe is suitable for Phase 1 to Phase 4.

Serving Size: 1

Time: 10 minutes

Prep Time: 10 minutes

Cook Time: N/A

Nutritional Facts/Info:

- Calories 163
- Net Carbs 1.3 g
- Fiber 0.3 g
- Sugars 1 g
- Fat 11.2 g
- Protein 13.4 g

Ingredients:

- 2 oz smoked salmon — shredded
- 2 tbsp feta cheese — crumbled
- ¼ cup lettuce — shredded
- ¼ cup baby spinach — shredded
- 2 tbsp watercress — shredded
- 1 tbsp white wine vinegar
- 1 tsp olive oil
- 1 tsp Stevia or sweetener on the approved list

Directions:

1. In a bowl, mix together the white wine vinegar, olive oil, and Stevia.

2. Shake the dress well so all the mixture combines.

3. In a salad bowl, mix together the lettuce, baby spinach, and watercress.

4. Add the smoked salmon and gently work it into the salad leaves.

5. Add the feta cheese.

6. Drizzle with the olive oil and vinegar salad dressing.

Recipe 12 — Hearty Cream of Asparagus Soup

This recipe can be enjoyed all year long. It can be used as a lunch or dinner recipe and can be complemented with pumpkin seeds for Phase 2 of the Atkins diet.

The recipe is suitable for Phase 1 to Phase 4.

Serving Size: 4 portions

Time: 55 minutes

Prep Time: 25 minutes

Cook Time: 30 minutes

Nutritional Facts/Info:

- Calories 93
- Net Carbs 4.7 g
- Fiber 2.8 g
- Sugars 3.9 g
- Fat 5 g
- Protein 6 g

Ingredients:

- 1 lb asparagus — chopped
- 2 celery stalks — chopped
- ½ red onion — chopped into large chunks
- 21.5 oz vegetable broth
- ½ cup cream — heavy
- dash of salt
- black pepper to taste
- 2 tsp coconut oil or vegetable oil

Directions:

1. In a large saucepan, heat the coconut or vegetable oil.
2. Place the onions into the saucepan and cook until soft and glassy.
3. Add the celery and asparagus to the saucepan.
4. Add the salt and slowly pour in the vegetable broth.
5. Bring the mixture to a slow boil, then turn the heat down to a simmer.
6. Cover the saucepan and allow the soup to simmer gently for 20 minutes.
7. After 20 minutes, remove the soup from the stove and allow it to cool down for 10 minutes.
8. When the soup has cooled down to warm, pour it into a blender and purée.
9. When the soup is smooth, pour it back into the saucepan, add the cream, some salt, and pepper to taste.
10. Heat on medium heat for another 10 minutes until the soup is piping hot.
11. Remove from the stove, add to soup bowls, and enjoy.

Recipe 13 — Low-Carb Cheesy Sausage and Mushroom Pizza

When you move to Phase 2 and 3, you can enjoy more foods, like low-carb pizza with flour basses. This is a pizza that you can enjoy from Phase 1 and has a cauliflower base.

This recipe can also be used as a dinner recipe.

The recipe is suitable for Phase 1 to Phase 4.

Serving Size: 4 pieces of pizza

Time: 55 minutes

Prep Time: 10 minutes

Cook Time: 45 minutes

Nutritional Facts/Info:

- Calories 53
- Net Carbs 4.6 g
- Fiber 1.5 g
- Sugars 3 g
- Fat 2.5 g
- Protein 2.8 g

Ingredients:

- 1 egg
- ½ small white onion — chopped
- ½ red bell pepper — chopped
- 1 cauliflower head — medium (must be equivalent to 3 cups)
- 1 tbsp pitted sliced black olives
- 1 tbsp pitted sliced green olives

- 1 cup mozzarella cheese — shredded

- 1 cup Parmesan cheese — shredded

- 2 tbsp tomato paste — unsweetened, organic

- ¼ tsp cayenne pepper

- ¼ tsp garlic salt

- ¼ tsp Italian spice

Directions:

1. Preheat the oven to 435° F.
2. Boil the cauliflower on the stove or in the microwave until it is soft enough to mash.
3. When the cauliflower is cooked, let it cool down for 10 to 15 minutes.
4. When the cauliflower is cool, squeeze out any excess water from the vegetable.
5. Mash the base together with the Parmesan cheese.
6. Fold the egg into the mixture and add the Italian spice, the cayenne pepper, and garlic salt.
7. Make the mixture into a tight ball.
8. Cut parchment paper to fit a 9-inch round pizza or pie dish.
9. Place the parchment in the round dish.
10. Put the cauliflower dough into the dish and form it into a round pizza base. It should be about ¼ inch thick.
11. Place the cauliflower pizza base into the pre-heated oven for 18 to 20 minutes. Turn the base half-way through the baking process to ensure both sides cook evenly.
12. When the crust is a nice golden brown, remove it from the oven and let it cool for five minutes.
13. When the crust is cool enough to touch, spread the tomato paste on the base.
14. Top with the finely chopped onion, bell pepper, and olives.
15. Spread the mozzarella cheese over the top.
16. Place the pizza back into the oven to bake for another 8 to 10 minutes.
17. When the pizza is cooked through, remove it from the oven and let it cool for 2 to 5 minutes.

18. Cut the pizza into 4 slices and serve.

Recipe 14 — Portobello Chicken Burger With Feta and Shallots

You can swap the chicken out for beef or turkey in this recipe.

From Phase 2, you can add 1 slice of tomato (0.4 g net carbs) to the burger and ½ a dill pickle (0.3 g net carbs). Remember to keep an eye on your carb count.

The recipe is suitable for Phase 1 to Phase 4.

Serving Size: 1

Time: 25 minutes

Prep Time: 10 minutes

Cook Time: 15 minutes

Nutritional Facts/Info:

- Calories 132
- Net Carbs 1.8 g
- Fiber 0.5 g
- Sugars 0.8 g
- Fat 7.5 g
- Protein 13.8 g

Ingredients:

- 2 oz chicken — minced
- 2 medium portobello mushrooms — remove the stalk
- 1 tsp shallots — chopped
- 2 tbsp feta cheese — crumbled
- black pepper to taste
- 1 tsp coconut oil or vegetable oil

250

Directions:

1. Add the chopped shallots, 1 tbsp crumbled feta cheese, and pepper to taste to the minced chicken.

2. Work the chicken into a burger patty shape.

3. In a skillet, heat the coconut or vegetable oil.

4. Cook the chicken burger patty until it is cooked through.

5. Top each of the portobello mushrooms with ½ tbsp feta cheese.

6. Heat the grill and add the two portobello mushrooms.

7. Grill the mushrooms until warm and slightly soft.

8. Remove the mushrooms from the grill.

9. Place the chicken burger patty on one of the mushrooms.

10. Cover the top of the burger with the other mushroom.

CHAPTER 11: LOW-CARB DINNER RECIPES

Here are 7 easy-to-make low-carb dinner recipes.

Please note that the nutritional information is per serving and that the carbohydrates reflect the **net carbs** and **not** the total carbs.

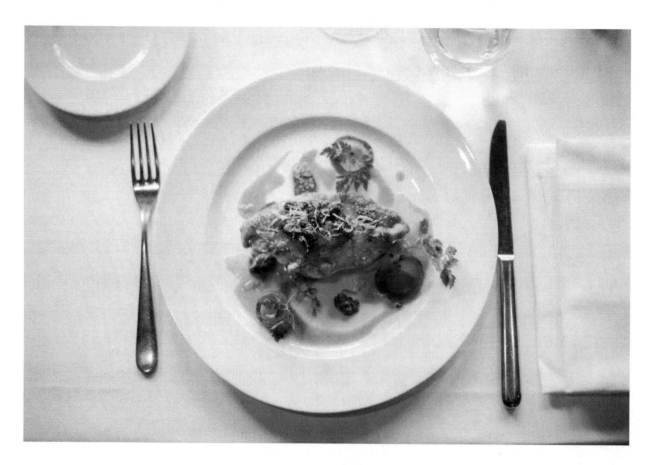

Recipe 15 — Beef Stroganoff on a Bed of Green Beans

This is a simple and easy-to-cook low-carb beef stroganoff that is complemented by the taste of the green beans.

The recipe is suitable for Phase 2 to Phase 4.

Serving Size: 2

Time: 30 minutes

Prep Time: 10 minutes

Cook Time: 20 minutes

Nutritional Facts/Info:

- Calories 167
- Net Carbs 7.5 g
- Fiber 3.2 g
- Sugars 3 g
- Fat 7.6 g
- Protein 3 g

Ingredients:

- 2 oz stir fry beef
- 1 cup brown mushrooms — halved
- ½ white onion — chopped
- 1 cup green beans — fresh and halved
- ½ cup beef broth
- ¼ glass of red wine
- 2 tbsp cream — soured
- salt and black pepper to taste

- 1 tsp mustard powder

- 1 tbsp coconut or vegetable oil

- ½ tbsp of butter — unsalted

Directions:

1. Heat the oil in a saucepan on medium heat.

2. Brown the meat and onion.

3. When the meat has been seared and the onion is glassy, remove the ingredients from the saucepan. Put them to one side.

4. Using the same saucepan, melt the butter, add the mushrooms, and sauté until they are soft but still firm.

5. Add the wine and beef broth to the mushrooms.

6. Allow the mixture to simmer on medium heat for 8 to 10 minutes.

7. While the mixture is simmering, cook the green beans in a saucepan of water over medium heat.

8. When the beans are soft but firm, remove from the stove and drain off excess water.

9. Add a bit of black pepper to taste and put them in a warmer drawer.

10. After 8 to 10 minutes, add the meat mixture and stir in well.

11. Slowly pour in the sour cream, stirring as you pour it into the mixture.

12. Turn the stove down to a heat that allows the stroganoff to simmer gently.

13. Allow the mixture to simmer for a further 3 to 5 minutes.

14. When the mixture is cooked, remove from the heat.

15. Add salt and pepper to taste.

16. Dish the green beans into two bowls.

17. Top the green beans with the beef stroganoff and serve while hot.

Recipe 16 — Fillet Medallions With Blackberry, Feta, and Spinach Salad

In Phase 2 of the Atkins diet, you can start to enjoy fruits and berries. This steak salad bursts with flavor with the mix of blackberries and feta.

The recipe is suitable for Phase 2 to Phase 4.

Serving Size: 1

Time: 25 minutes

Prep Time: 10 minutes

Cook Time: 15 minutes

Nutritional Facts/Info:

- Calories 361
- Net Carbs 6.3 g
- Fiber 2 g
- Sugars 3 g
- Fat 28.7 g
- Protein 19.6 g

Ingredients:

- 2 oz beef fillet steak — cut into 1-inch medallions
- 2 tbsp blackberries — halved
- ¼ baby spinach leaves — shredded
- 2 tbsp arugula
- 2 tbsp feta cheese — crumbled
- 1 tbsp fresh basil
- 1 tsp roasted sesame seeds (optional)
- 1 tbsp mayonnaise

- 1 tsp mustard powder

- 1 tsp stevia or sweetener of your choice on the approved foods list

- ½ tsp tomato sauce

- 2 tsp coconut oil or vegetable oil

Directions:

1. In a large skillet, heat the coconut or vegetable oil

2. Cook the fillet medallions to your liking.

3. When the steak is cooked, remove it from the heat and put it to one side to cool.

4. In a salad bowl, mix the arugula, baby spinach leaves, and basil.

5. In a jar or jug, mix together the mayonnaise, mustard powder, tomato sauce, and Stevia. You can add a dash of white wine vinegar to give it an extra tang and make the mixture a little runny.

6. When the steak has cooled down, mix it into the salad bowl.

7. Add the blackberries, sesame seeds, and crumbled feta cheese.

8. Drizzle the mayonnaise dressing over it — try the salad with just a bit of pepper first as you may not like the mayonnaise dressing mix with the berries.

Recipe 17 — Lamb Chops With Cauliflower Mash

Lamb chops work well with mashed cauliflower and a bit of Dijon mustard.

The recipe is suitable for Phase 1 to Phase 4.

Serving Size: 1

Time: 25 minutes

Prep Time: 10 minutes

Cook Time: 15 minutes

Nutritional Facts/Info:

- Calories 478
- Net Carbs 5.6 g
- Fiber 6.2 g
- Sugars 1.2 g
- Fat 37.1 g
- Protein 26.5 g

Ingredients:

- 1 lamb chop
- ½ cup cauliflower
- 4 cherry tomatoes — halved
- ¼ cup brown mushrooms — halved
- ¼ avocado
- 2 tsp coconut oil
- 2 tsp Dijon mustard
- 2 tsp unsalted butter
- 1 tsp rosemary — fresh (crushed) or dried
- 1 ¼ tsp salt
- 1 ¼ tsp black pepper

Directions:

1. Boil the cauliflower in a saucepan of water until soft enough to mash.
2. When the cauliflower is done, drain off all excess water.
3. Add ¼ tsp of salt and ¼ black pepper to flavor. You do not have to use all of the designated amounts of salt or pepper; season to your taste.
4. While the cauliflower is cooking, rub each of the lamb chops with a bit of coconut oil and Dijon mustard.

5. Mix 1 tsp black pepper, 1 tsp salt, and 1 tsp rosemary on a dinner plate.

6. Dip the lamb chop rubbed with coconut oil onto the rosemary mix. Do both sides of the chop to coat them with the rosemary mix.

7. Put the lamb chop into a grilling/baking dish and place under the grill until cooked to your liking.

8. About 2 minutes before the chop is ready to come off the grill, add the mushrooms and cherry tomatoes.

9. Dish the cauliflower mash onto a plate.

10. Top the cauliflower mash with the lamb chop, grilled tomato, and mushrooms.

11. Slice the ¼ avocado in long medium-thick slices and serve with the dish.

Recipe 18 — Cauliflower and Minced Beef Fritters

You can use cauliflower with minced beef to make tasty beef fritters.

The recipe is suitable for Phase 2 to Phase 4.

Serving Size: 6 fritters

Time: 25 minutes

Prep Time: 10 minutes

Cook Time: 15 minutes

Nutritional Facts/Info:

- Calories 142
- Net Carbs 2 g
- Fiber 1.2 g
- Sugars 0.4 g
- Fat 9.4 g
- Protein 12.2 g

Ingredients:

- 1 egg
- 3 oz ground beef
- ½ cup cauliflower — mashed
- 1 tbsp shallots — finely chopped
- 1 cup iceberg lettuce — shredded
- 2 tbsp fresh basil — shredded
- ¼ cup arugula — shredded
- 2 tbsp almond flour — blanched
- 2 tsp coconut oil or vegetable oil
- 1 tsp mixed herb spice
- dash of black pepper to taste

Directions:

1. Cook and mash the cauliflower.
2. In a mixing bowl, mix the ground beef and cauliflower mash.
3. Fold the egg into the ground beef and cauliflower mixture.
4. Add the finely chopped shallots to the ground beef and cauliflower mixture.
5. Sift in the almond flour a bit at a time to firm the mixture.
6. Add the mixed herb spice and pepper to taste.
7. Divide the mixture up into 4 to 6 balls and flatten into 1.4-inch thick fritter rounds.
8. Heat the coconut oil in a skillet.
9. You should be able to cook at least 3 fritters at a time in the skillet.
10. When they are cooked, dish up onto a plate and serve on a bed of crisp shredded lettuce, arugula, and basil leaves.

Recipe 19 — Vegetable Lamb Stew

This hearty beef stew can be enjoyed as a dinner or lunch recipe.

The recipe is suitable for Phase 2 to Phase 4.

Serving Size: 2

Time: 1 hour and 20 minutes

Prep Time: 20 minutes

Cook Time: 1 hour

Nutritional Facts/Info:

- Calories 476
- Net Carbs 5.6 g
- Fiber 1.9 g
- Sugars 3.6 g
- Fat 22 g
- Protein 58.9 g

Ingredients:

- 14 oz lamb — cubed
- ¼ cup turnip
- ¼ cup cauliflower
- ¼ brussels sprouts
- 1 white onion — chopped
- 1 garlic clove — crushed
- 6.7 fl. oz vegetable broth
- 2 tsp fresh basil
- 2 tbsp vegetable oil
- pepper to taste

Directions:

1. Heat 1 tsp of vegetable oil in a medium pot over medium heat.

2. Add chopped onions and cook until glassy.

3. Remove onions from the pot and put them to one side.

4. Add 1 tsp of vegetable oil to the pot you removed the onions from.

5. Brown lamb cubes in the heated oil.

6. Add the chopped turnip, cauliflower, and brussels sprouts.

7. Add the vegetable stock and cooked onions to the ingredients in the pot.

8. Bring to a boil and then turn the heat down to allow the stew to simmer.

9. Add the crushed garlic clove, basil, and season to taste.

10. Cover the stew and allow it to simmer gently for 1 hour or until the meat and vegetables are soft.

11. Dish into bowls and serve hot.

Recipe 20 — Simple Vegetable Beef Chili

This warm chili can be adjusted to suit how spicy you want it to be. For this recipe, the chili is mild to medium spiced.

The recipe is suitable for Phase 1 to Phase 4.

Serving Size: 2

Time: 35 minutes

Prep Time: 10 minutes

Cook Time: 25 minutes

Nutritional Facts/Info:

- Calories 436
- Net Carbs 3.9 g
- Fiber 5 g
- Sugars 4.4 g
- Fat 24 g
- Protein 30 g

Ingredients:

- 3 oz ground beef
- 1 cup brown mushrooms — halved
- ¼ cup zucchini — chopped into bite-sized chunks
- ¼ cup pumpkin — bite-sized cubes
- 1 tsp garlic — crushed
- 2 tbsp cream — heavy
- ¼ cup beef broth
- 2 tsp chili powder — mild to medium
- 1 tsp black pepper
- 1 tsp mixed herbs spice
- 1 tsp coconut oil or vegetable oil

Directions:

1. On the stove or in the microwave, cook the chopped zucchini until it is firm but starting to get soft.
2. Drain all excess water off the zucchini once it is done and put it to one side.
3. On the stove or in the microwave, cook the cubed pumpkin until it is firm but starting to get soft.
4. Drain all the excess water off the pumpkin once it is done and put it to one side.

5. Heat oil in a saucepan.

6. Add ground beef and crushed garlic.

7. Flavor the ground beef with mixed herbs and black pepper.

8. When the ground beef is browned, add the mushrooms, semi-cooked zucchini, and pumpkin.

9. Add the beef broth, chili powder, and pepper to taste.

10. Bring the mixture to a boil stirring it regularly.

11. Turn the chili down to low heat and allow it to simmer for 10 minutes to allow the flavor to set and the vegetable to soften.

12. After 10 minute stir in the cream.

13. Allow the mixture to simmer for a further 5 minutes before removing from heat.

14. Dish into bowls and serve piping hot.

Recipe 21 — Chicken Breast Stuffed With Goat Cheese and Asparagus

This dish can be used for a lunch recipe as well. It can be served hot or cold.

You do not have to use the mustard mayonnaise sauce if you do not wish to.

The recipe is suitable for Phase 1 to Phase 4.

Serving Size: 2

Time: 53 minutes

Prep Time: 15 minutes

Cook Time: 38 minutes

Nutritional Facts/Info:

- Calories 296
- Net Carbs 3 g
- Fiber 1.5 g
- Sugars 2 g
- Fat 14.3 g
- Protein 36.2 g

Ingredients:

- 2 x 4 oz lean chicken breasts
- 6 large asparagus stalks — halved
- ¼ brown mushrooms — halved
- 1 tsp dill — finely chopped
- 1 tbsp goat cheese — semi-soft
- ¼ tsp garlic — crushed
- 1 tsp butter
- 2 tsp mayonnaise
- cayenne or black pepper to taste
- ¼ tsp mustard powder

Directions:

1. Preheat the oven to 350° F.
2. Cut each chicken breast in half but be careful not to cut all the way through. You are going to put the stuffing on one half and pull the other half over it when the chicken has been cooked.
3. Grease a casserole or baking pan.
4. Place the 2 cut-open chicken breasts in the dish/pan and place them in the oven.

5. Bake for approximately 25 to 30 minutes, turning the chicken over halfway through baking.

6. When there are 15 minutes left for the cooking of the chicken, start preparation on the filling and the sauce.

7. In a saucepan or microwaveable bowl, place the halved asparagus spears and mushrooms.

8. Add a dash of black pepper and crushed garlic.

9. If you are cooking on the stove, heat the ingredients until the butter has melted. The asparagus and mushrooms should be soft but still slightly firm.

10. Drain off excess butter.

11. When the chicken is cooked, remove it from the oven.

12. Add the cooked mushrooms and asparagus to the one-half of each of the chicken breasts.

13. Crumble goat cheese over the mushroom and asparagus filling.

14. Place half of the chicken breast without the filling over the top of the mixture.

15. Put the stuffed chicken breasts back into the oven and back for another 5 to 8 minutes, or until the goat cheese has melted.

16. While the chicken is baking, in a mixing bowl, mix together the mayonnaise and mustard powder.

17. When the chicken breasts are done, remove them from the oven.

18. Serve them on a dinner plate, topped with a dollop of mustard mayonnaise sauce, a dash of cayenne pepper, and a sprinkling of freshly chopped dill.

CHAPTER 12: LOW-CARB RECIPES FOR THE SWEET TOOTH

Here are 7 easy-to-make low-carb desserts or baked goods.

Please note that the nutritional information is per serving and that the carbohydrates reflect the **net carbs** and **not** the total carbs.

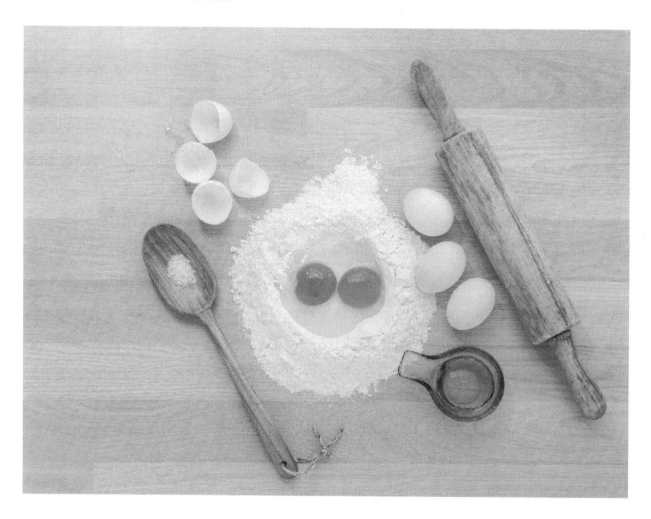

Recipe 22 — Bite-Sized Salted Caramel No-Bake Cheesecake Blocks

This delicious low-carb treat has under 1 g of net carbs per bite-sized block..

The recipe is suitable for Phase 2 to Phase 4.

Serving Size: 9 bite-sized blocks

Time: 1 hour 45 minutes

Prep Time: 15 minutes

Setting Time: 1 hour 30 minutes

Nutritional Facts/Info:

- Calories 66
- Net Carbs 0.9 g
- Fiber 3.1 g
- Sugars 0.3 g
- Fat 6.3 g
- Protein 1.9 g

Ingredients:

- ¼ cup macadamia nuts — crushed/bits
- ¼ tsp xanthan gum
- ¼ cup whey protein — unflavored or vanilla flavor can be used
- 3 tsp Stevia — sugar form and not the liquid
- 2 pinches of salt — up to ¼ tsp can be used
- 3 oz cream cheese
- ¼ cream — heavy
- 2 tsp caramel syrup — sugar-free
- ½ tsp vanilla extract

Directions:

1. Use a freezer-safe tray, approximately 7" w x 1.5" l x 1.5" deep.

2. Cut a piece of parchment paper big enough to cover the base and sides of the dish.

3. Place the parchment paper into the dish and put it to one side.

4. You can use an ice cube tray (lightly grease it) or freezer-safe silicone mold.

5. Whisk together the cream cheese, vanilla extract, 1 pinch of salt, and caramel syrup in a large mixing bowl.

6. Add the macadamia nuts, mixing them thoroughly into the mixture.

7. In another mixing bowl, mix the whey protein powder and cream until the mixture is smooth.

8. Fold the whey protein and cream mixture into the cream cheese mix, blend the mixture in a blender until smooth.

9. Add the xanthan gum and blend the mixture for another minute.

10. Pour the mixture into the freezer-safe dish.

11. Top with a light dash of salt.

12. Cover the mixture with plastic wrap.

13. Place the mixture in the freezer to set for 1 hour 30 minutes.

14. When the mixture has set, remove it from the freezer and cut into squares approximately 1-inch wide x ½-inch long.

Recipe 23 — Creamy Chocolate and Avocado Pudding

If you love chocolate pudding, you are going to love these low-carb chocolate and avocado pudding cups.

The recipe is suitable for Phase 2 to Phase 4.

Serving Size: 2

Time: 1 hour 15 minutes

Prep Time: 15 minutes

Setting Time: 1 hour

Nutritional Facts/Info:

- Calories 175
- Net Carbs 7 g
- Fiber 18.2 g
- Sugars 1.3 g
- Fat 7.2 g
- Protein 15.8 g

Ingredients:

- 2 tbsp mashed avocado
- 3 tbsp whey protein powder — vanilla or unflavored
- 2 tsp Stevia or sweetener of your choice from the approved food list
- ¾ tsp xanthan gum
- ½ tbsp cacao powder — unsweetened
- ½ tsp vanilla extract

Directions:

1. In a mixing bowl, blend together the avocado, cream, and whey protein powder until smooth.

2. Add the cacao powder, vanilla, xanthan gum, and Stevia.

3. Blend the mixture together until smooth and creamy.

4. Divide the mixture into 2 fridge safe small pudding bowls or cups.

5. Cover each bowl with plastic wrap.

6. Place the bowls in the refrigerator for 1 hour to set before serving.

Recipe 24 — Spicy Dark Chocolate Chip Vanilla Cheesecake Pudding Cups

This is a quick and easy to make vanilla cheesecake pudding. It has a rich warm flavor of allspice blended with the unique flavor of dark chocolate chips.

The recipe is suitable for Phase 1 to Phase 4.

Serving Size: 3

Time: 1 hour and 35 minutes

Prep Time: 15 minutes

Setting Time: 1 hour and 20 minutes

Nutritional Facts/Info:

- Calories 179
- Net Carbs 3.1 g
- Fiber 0.4 g
- Sugars 1.5 g
- Fat 18.3 g
- Protein 2.6 g

Ingredients:

- 1 tbsp dark chocolate nibs — sugar-free
- 3 oz cream cheese
- 3 tbsp cream — heavy
- ½ tbsp sour cream
- 1 ½ tbsp Stevia — powder/sugar and not the liquid
- ½ tsp allspice
- ½ tsp vanilla extract

Directions:

1. Place 3 pudding cups or small bowls into the freezer before you start to bake.
2. In a mixing bowl, blend together 1 tbsp Stevia, the sour cream, cream, cheese, and all-spice.
3. Blend together on medium until the mixture is thick and smooth.
4. Add the vanilla extract and chocolate chips; mix well.
5. In another mixing bowl, blend the heavy cream and ½ tbsp of Stevia until the cream thickens and forms soft peaks.
6. Fold the thickened cream into the sour cream and cream cheese mixture until it is well mixed together.
7. Using the iced pudding bowls from the freezer, spoon the mixture evenly into the 3 pudding bowls.
8. Cover each one with plastic wrap.
9. Place them in the refrigerator for 2 hours to set before serving.

Recipe 25 — Berry Cherry Ice Pops

These flavored fruit and berry pops are quick and easy to make. They will help to stave off your sweet tooth, they are refreshing, and a nice quick summer snack.

The recipe is suitable for Phase 2 to Phase 4.

Serving Size: 6 ice pops

Time: 2 hours 10 minutes to 4 hours 10 minutes

Prep Time: 10 minutes

Setting Time: 2 to 4 hours

Nutritional Facts/Info:

- Calories 11
- Net Carbs 1.8 g
- Fiber 1 g
- Sugars 1.6 g
- Fat 0.1 g
- Protein 0.2 g

Ingredients:

- ¼ cup blackberries — fresh or unsweetened frozen
- ¼ cup raspberries — fresh or unsweetened frozen
- ¼ cup blueberries — fresh or unsweetened frozen
- ¼ cup strawberries — fresh or unsweetened frozen
- 4 tbsp cherry syrup — sugar-free (Atkins or Da Vinci)
- 1 tsp lemon zest
- 1 tsp lime zest
- 1 cup of filtered water

Directions:

1. Blend the berries together with the filtered water.

2. Add the cherry syrup, lemon zest, and lime zest.

3. Blend for 30 seconds.

4. You can add another tbsp of cherry syrup if you feel it necessary.

5. Pour into 6 ice pop molds.

6. Place in the freezer for 2 to 4 hours or until completely set.

Recipe 26 — Refreshing Caramel Fruit and Berry Salad

This fruit salad makes a nice addition to a meal for Phase 3 and Phase 4. You can use it as a meal or halve it for a snack in Phase 2.

The recipe is suitable for Phase 2 to Phase 4.

Serving Size: 1

Time: 15 minutes

Prep Time: 15 minutes

Cook Time: N/A

Nutritional Facts/Info:

- Calories 151
- Net Carbs 8.1 g
- Fiber 2.4 g
- Sugars 7.3 g
- Fat 11.9 g
- Protein 1 g

Ingredients:

- 1 tbsp blackberries — fresh or unsweetened frozen
- 1 tbsp raspberries — fresh or unsweetened frozen
- 1 tbsp blueberries — fresh or unsweetened frozen
- ¼ cup honeydew melon — balls
- 1 tsp mint leaves — fresh and shredded
- 2 mint leaves — fresh
- 2 tbsp cream — heavy
- 2 tsp sour cream
- 1 tbsp caramel syrup — sugar-free (Da Vinci) optional
- 1 tsp Stevia or sweetener of your choice

Directions:

1. Place the berries, shredded mint, and honeydew melon in a bowl.
2. Place the bowl in the freezer for 10 minutes.
3. In a mixing bowl, blend the heavy cream together with the Stevia until the cream forms soft peaks.
4. Fold in the sour and caramel syrup.
5. After 10 minutes, remove the fruit and berries from the freezer.
6. Top with cream mixture.
7. Garnish with the two mint leaves and enjoy.

Recipe 27 — Nutty Crust Pumpkin Pie

This pie can be enjoyed in Phase 3.

The recipe is suitable for Phase 3 to Phase 4.

Serving Size: 8 slices

Time: 65 minutes

Prep Time: 15 minutes

Cook Time: 50 minutes

Nutritional Facts/Info:

- Calories 258
- Net Carbs 6.5 g
- Fiber 2.4 g
- Sugars 4.8 g
- Fat 23.8 g
- Protein 3.5 g

Ingredients:

- 2 eggs — large and at room temperature
- 2 cups walnuts — ground
- 1 ½ cups cream — heavy
- 2 cups pumpkin, canned, without salt
- ¼ cup butter — unsalted and melted
- 1 tsp allspice
- ½ tsp pumpkin spice
- ½ cup Stevia or sweetener of your choice from the approved food list
- 2 tsp Stevia (for the walnut base)
- dash of salt

Directions:

1. Preheat the oven to 325° F.

2. Combine the ground walnuts, melted butter, and 2 tsp of Stevia in a mixing bowl.

3. Lightly grease a 9-inch pie dish.

4. Firmly press the nut mixture into the pie dish to form a pie crust shell.

5. Place in the oven and bake for 10 minutes or until the crust turns golden brown. Be careful not to burn it.

6. While the pie crust is baking, prepare the filling.

7. Whisk together ½ cup of Stevia or sugar substitute, allspice, pumpkin spice, canned pumpkin, and add a dash of salt.

8. In another mixing bowl, mix the heavy cream until it forms soft firm peaks.

9. Fold the cream into the pumpkin mixture.

10. Place plastic wrap over it and place it in the fridge while the pie crust cools.

11. Remove the walnut crust pie shell from the oven and allow it to cool for 5 to 10 minutes.

12. Increase the heat of the oven to 375° F.

13. When the pie crust has cooled, take the pumpkin mixture out of the refrigerator and scoop it into the pie crust.

14. Distribute the mixture evenly.

15. Place the pie in the oven and bake for 30 to 40 minutes.

16. The middle of the pie should be nice and wobbly.

17. Cut into 6 pieces and serve.

Recipe 28 — Peppermint Chocolate Mousse

This minty chocolate mousse can be enjoyed from Phase 1.

The recipe is suitable for Phase 1 to Phase 4.

Serving Size: 3

Time: 1 hour and 15 minutes

Prep Time: 15 minutes

Setting Time: 1 hour

Nutritional Facts/Info:

- Calories 268
- Net Carbs 6.1g
- Fiber 0.9 g
- Sugars 6.3 g
- Fat 22.5 g
- Protein 8.5 g

Ingredients:

- 1 ½ scoop of whey protein — vanilla flavor
- 1 tsp cocoa powder — raw organic unsweetened
- 1 cups of cream — heavy
- 6 fresh mint leaves
- 1 tbsp Stevia or sweetener of your choice from the approved foods list
- ¼ tsp mint extract

Directions:

1. Place 3 pudding bowls in the freezer for 10 minutes.

2. Shred 4 of the fresh mint leaves and put the remaining two aside.

3. In a blender, beat the cream into soft stiff peaks.

4. Fold in the whey protein powder, cocoa powder, Stevia, shredded mint leaves, and peppermint extract.

5. Beat the ingredients until thick.

6. Remove the bowls from the freezer.

7. Scoop the mousse evenly into the 3 dessert bowls.

8. Cover each bowl with plastic wrap and place in the refrigerator.

9. Allow the mousse to set for at least 1 hour.

10. Remove from the refrigerator when the mousse has set and enjoy.

CHAPTER 13: DELICIOUS LOW-CARB SMOOTHIES AND BEVERAGES

Here are 7 easy-to-make low-carb smoothies.

Please note that the nutritional information is per serving and that the carbohydrates reflect the **net carbs** and **not** the total carbs.

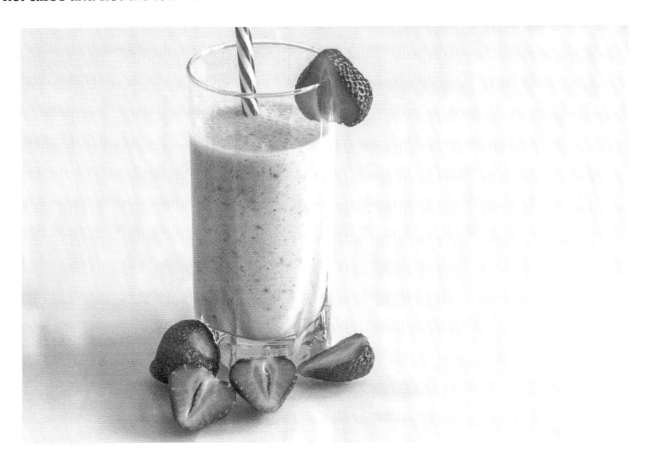

Recipe 29 — Peanut Butter Smoothie

Anyone who loves peanut butter is probably going to miss the peanut butter sandwiches as you are not able to eat bread, especially during the first few phases of the diet. This smoothie will satisfy both your hunger pangs and peanut butter cravings.

If you like eating peanut butter and celery, you can add 1 medium-sized chopped celery stalk to the recipe (0.2 net carbs).

You can use ¼ cup of coconut milk (2 g net carbs) instead of almond milk (0.3 g net carbs).

The recipe is suitable for Phase 1 to Phase 4.

Serving Size: 1

Time: 10 minutes

Prep Time: 10 minutes

Cook Time: N/A

Nutritional Facts/Info:

- Calories 292
- Net Carbs 6.1 g
- Fiber 3.4g
- Sugars 2.9 g
- Fat 21.4 g
- Protein 17.6 g

Ingredients:

- ½ cup of filtered water
- ½ cup almond milk — unsweetened, always choose the organic option if possible
- ½ tablespoon cocoa powder — unsweetened, the organic one is preferable

- 1 scoop whey protein powder — vanilla or chocolate flavor
- 2 tbsp peanut butter — smooth with no added sugar or salt
- 1 tsp/packet of Stevia sweetener or your preferred choice from the approved foods list
- ½ tsp vanilla extract
- ¼ tsp nutmeg

Directions:

1. In a blender or smoothie mixer, add the coconut milk, whey protein powder, water, and cocoa powder.
2. Blend together thoroughly.
3. Add peanut butter, vanilla, nutmeg, and Stevia.
4. Blend ingredients together thoroughly.
5. Pour into a glass or a sealed drinking flask/container.

Recipe 30 — Raspberry Coconut Zinger Smoothie

This smoothie comes with a bit of a bite as you add cayenne pepper and ginger.

You can use ¼ cup of coconut milk instead of ¼ almond milk; coconut milk is a lot higher in net carbs than almond milk.

The recipe is suitable for Phase 2 up to Phase 4.

Serving Size: 1

Time: 10 minutes

Prep Time: 10 minutes

Cook Time: N/A

Nutritional Facts/Info:

- Calories 189
- Net Carbs 6.1 g
- Fiber 4.5 g
- Sugars 3 g
- Fat 9 g
- Protein 19.6 g

Ingredients:

- 2 tbsp raspberries — fresh if possible, for frozen they must be unsweetened
- 1 tbsp shaved coconut — unsweetened
- ½ cup of filtered water
- ¼ cup almond milk — unsweetened and if possible look for organic
- 1 scoop protein whey powder — vanilla flavored
- ½ tsp cinnamon
- ½ tsp ground ginger
- ¼ tsp cayenne pepper

Directions:

1. Add all the ingredients into a blender or smoothie mixer.
2. Blend together thoroughly.
3. Pour into a glass or into a sealed drinking flask/container.

Recipe 31 — Blackberry Pecan Pie Smoothie

You can use ½ cup of coconut milk instead of ½ cup almond milk; remember to watch the net carbs as coconut milk is higher in carbs.

The recipe is suitable for Phase 2 to Phase 4.

Serving Size: 1

Time: 10 minutes

Prep Time: 10 minutes

Cook Time: N/A

Nutritional Facts/Info:

- Calories 164
- Net Carbs 4.9 g
- Fiber 3 g
- Sugars 2 g
- Fat 3.2 g
- Protein 8.6 g

Ingredients:

- 10 pecans
- 2 tbsp blackberries — fresh if possible, or unsweetened frozen
- ½ cup of filtered water
- ½ cup almond milk — unsweetened
- 1 scoop of whey protein powder — chocolate
- 2 tsp Stevia sweetener or a sweetener of your choice
- 3 tsp sugar-free maple syrup

Directions:

1. Add all the ingredients into a blender or smoothie mixer.

2. Blend together thoroughly.

3. Pour into a glass or into a sealed drinking flask/container.

Recipe 32 — Chocolate, Mint, and Avocado Smoothie

This smoothie can be enjoyed as a snack or a meal replacement.

You can add an optional 1 tsp of fresh basil to give it a unique flavor. You can also add a dash of cayenne pepper to get your metabolism going in the morning and give you some zing.

You can use 1 cup almond milk instead of 1 cup of coconut milk; you will need to adjust the net carb amount as coconut milk is higher in carbs than almond milk.

The recipe is suitable for Phase 1 to Phase 4.

Serving Size: 1

Time: 10 minutes

Prep Time: 10 minutes

Cook Time: N/A

Nutritional Facts/Info:

- Calories 209
- Net Carbs 5.7 g
- Fiber 4.6 g
- Sugars 1.7 g
- Fat 13.3 g
- Protein 14.2 g

Ingredients:

- ¼ avocado

- 1 tbsp (½ scoop) whey protein powder — chocolate

- 1 tsp fresh mint

- ¼ glass of filtered water

- ¼ cup coconut milk, unsweetened

- ¼ tsp vanilla extract

- ½ cinnamon

Directions:

1. Cut the avocado into cubes

2. In a blender, mix together all the ingredients.

3. Pour into a glass and enjoy it.

Recipe 33 — Ginger, Cranberry, Cucumber, and Mint Fizz

This is a nice refreshing drink to top up with during a meal or after a workout.

Enjoy this drink over a glass of crushed ice after a long hot day in the sun.

The recipe is suitable for Phase 1 to Phase 4.

Serving Size: 1

Time: 10 minutes

Prep Time: 10 minutes

Cook Time: N/A

Nutritional Facts/Info:

- Calories 20

- Net Carbs 2.1 g

- Fiber 0.7 g

- Sugars 0.5 g

- Fat 1.2 g

- Protein 0.4 g

Ingredients:

- 1 tbsp cranberries

- 2 tbsp cucumber — finely chopped

- 1 tsp ginger — fresh, grated

- 1 tbsp mint — fresh shredded

- 1 cup club soda

- 1 tsp Stevia or sweetener of choice from the approved foods list.

Directions:

1. Add all the ingredients into a blender.

2. Blend together thoroughly.

3. Pour into a glass and enjoy it.

Recipe 34 — Lemon and Lime Raspberry Watermelon Fizz

This drink can be enjoyed both fizzy and still by replacing the club soda with still water. Enjoy this drink over a few blocks of ice in the summer.

The recipe is suitable for Phase 2 to Phase 4.

Serving Size: 1

Time: 10 minutes

Prep Time: 10 minutes

Cook Time: N/A

Nutritional Facts/Info:

- Calories 32
- Net Carbs 6.8 g
- Fiber 2.8 g
- Sugars 3.2 g
- Fat 0.3 g
- Protein 0.8 g

Ingredients:

- ½ lime — peeled, remove pips, and chop into small chunks
- ½ lemon — peeled, remove pips, and chop into small chunks
- 2 tbsp watermelon — remove the rind, remove pips, and cut into cubes
- 2 tbsp raspberries — fresh, or unsweetened frozen
- 2 tsp Stevia or sweetener of your choice from the approved foods list.

Directions:

1. Add all the ingredients into a blender.
2. Blend together thoroughly.
3. Pour into a glass and enjoy it.

Recipe 35 — Salted Caramel Iced Coffee

If you have a sweet tooth, you can substitute one of your meals for this decadent low-carb smoothie.

You can swap the almond milk out for coconut milk if you want to; just remember to re-calculate the net carbs for the recipe.

The recipe is suitable for Phase 1 to Phase 4.

Serving Size: 1

Time: 10 minutes

Prep Time: 10 minutes

Cook Time: N/A

Nutritional Facts/Info:

- Calories 165
- Net Carbs 3.1 g
- Fiber 1 g
- Sugars 0.1 g
- Fat 4.9 g
- Protein 23.3 g

Ingredients:

- 1 scoop whey protein — chocolate flavor
- 2 tbsp cream cheese — fat-free
- 1 cup almond milk — unsweetened, organic if possible
- 2 tsp caramel syrup — sugar-free
- ½ tsp salt (you can add up to 1 tsp if desired)
- 1 tsp fine coffee powder — decaffeinated is the best choice
- ¼ cup crushed ice

Directions:

1. Add all the ingredients, except for the crushed ice, into a blender or smoothie mixer.

2. Blend together thoroughly.

3. Pour the crushed ice into a glass.

4. Pour the smoothie over the crushed ice and enjoy it.

CHAPTER 14: ADDITIONAL RESOURCES FOR CONTINUED SUCCESS ON THE ATKINS DIET

The Atkins website has a whole host of online resources that includes articles, tips, ticks, recipes, and products.

You can find additional Atkins resources, recipes, and products online. I have highlighted some of the most useful pages on the site for you below.

About the Atkins Diet and the History

To learn more about the Atkins Diet, the history, and why a low-carb diet promotes weight loss, the following link will give you access to the "Our Story" page on the Atkins Website:

https://www.atkins.com/our-mission

Articles, Blogs, and Helpful Information

For articles, references, success stories, and more information on the Atkins Diet, the following link will take you to the Atkins blog page.

https://www.atkins.com/how-it-works/atkins-blogs

Atkins Healthcare Professional Portal

The Atkins Healthcare Professional Portal is mainly accessed by healthcare professionals but you can find some information about the science behind the diet. You can also find some useful and informative articles. You can access the portal from the following link:

http://www.atkins-hcp.com/

Products

Atkins offers a lot of great low-carb nutritious and delicious products. These products include:

- Atkins bars
- Atkins Shakes
- Atkins Treats
- Atkins Frozen Food & Meals

The snack, treats, and shakes are a great way to stave off your sweet tooth and they can be used in various recipes that Atkins provides.

Another great product from Atkins is their frozen foods and meals. They are great time savers and you know you are getting a good nutritious meal.

When you access the products page, Atkins has a handy nearest store finder where you type in your zip code and it will direct you to the nearest stockist of Atkins products.

You can access the Atkins products page from the following link:

https://www.atkins.com/products

Recipes

The Atkins website is filled with low-carb recipes that have a convenient search facility that lets you search by recipe phase, meal type, or recipe name.

Each recipe will specify what phase the recipe is suited for and comes with a nutrition table. You can access the Atkins recipes page by following the link below:

https://www.atkins.com/recipes

Success Stories

You can read some heartwarming and encouraging Atkins Diet success stories at the following link:

https://www.atkins.com/success-stories

WOULD YOU DO ME A SMALL FOVOR?

Thank you for reading this book. I hope you'll use what you've learned to look, feel and live better than you ever have before.

I have a small favor to ask.

Would you mind taking a minute to write a blurb on Amazon about this book? I check all my reviews and love to get honest feedback. That's the real pay for my work – knowing that I'm helping people.

Thanks again, and I really look forward to reading your feedback!

To post your review scan with your camera:

CONCLUSION

The Atkins Diet is not just a diet but a way of life. If you are serious about losing weight, getting healthy, and keeping the weight off, you need it to become your new lifestyle. When you start the diet, start thinking of the Atkins Diet as a lifetime commitment to a healthier, happier, and trimmer you. It may start off as a diet but it does not stop after the initial two to four weeks as it unfolds into a healthy eating plan.

Phase 1, the Inductions Phase, may seem pretty tough at first glance, but as you get into it, you will find there is a large variety of everyday foods to choose from. Play around with different recipes you find and make your own. Break out of your current comfort zone and let your taste buds expand their culinary horizons. A diet does not have to be boring; find the color and bring the choices you do have to life.

Phase 2 is the Continued Weight Loss Phase, which ups your carbs a bit and throws in some more foods you can eat. By the time you get to this phase, you will already be adding those carbs up in your head and designing your own low-carb dishes. Even if you are not a great cook, check out the easy-to-follow recipes included in this book and reinvent them.

Phase 3 is the Pre-Maintenance Phase. At this stage, you're at the border of reaching your goal weight. You are getting ready to step out of the diet mode into maintenance mode. This is the phase where you will start to learn how to manage your weight and food so you can confidently progress into the next stage.

Phase 4 is the Maintenance or Lifestyle Phase. This is the stage where you are ready to leave the Atkins Diet nest and take your first solo flight into the Atkins Lifestyle. Join various Atkins Diet support groups and newsletters. Keeping up with the dieting and eating trends is an important part of changing to a healthier lifestyle. There are always new developments and foods that all help you maintain your new lifestyle.

Exercise complements your weight loss regimen and will help to firm and tone your body. Exercise also offers health benefits and boosts your self-confidence. Just don't overdo the exercise.

Use the meal plans and acceptable food lists from the chapters above to make quick and easy grocery lists. Fill up on water or at least have a low-carb snack before you go do your grocery shopping to stop cravings and filling up on junk food high in carbs.

Don't get despondent if you have off-days or slip-ups; take them as they come, forgive yourself for them, and move on. Most importantly, remember not to give up, keep pushing through. Nothing is ever easy to begin with, but the end result is well worth the effort.

If you have made it to the end of the book and have started your Atkins lifestyle journey, well done.

As I love to hear from my readers, please leave a review and let me know how you enjoyed the book.

Enjoy the new healthier and slimmer you.

At **BODY YOU DESERVE Publishing**, we strongly believe that there are a thousand ways to improve your life and health. However, there is no single recipe suitable for everyone how to do that.

We think that the best way to receive your goals is the one you can stick to and our writers will do their best to provide simple, easy to follow, step by step and realistic instructions how to do that.

To discover our best books scan with your camera:

REFERENCES

Atkins for Vegans. (n.d.). Atkins. https://www.atkins-hcp.com/atkins-resources/research/atkins-for-vegans-1

Atkins for Veggies. (n.d.). Atkins. https://uk.atkins.com/blog/atkins-for-veggies/

Butler, N. (2020, January 30). *Atkins diet: What is it, and should I try it?* Medical News Today. https://www.medicalnewstoday.com/articles/7379

Carbohydrates. (n.d.). Cleveland Clinic. https://my.clevelandclinic.org/health/articles/15416-carbohydrates

Coyle, D. (2018, October 03). *Starchy vs Non-Starchy Vegetables: Food Lists and Nutrition Facts*. Healthline. https://www.healthline.com/nutrition/starchy-vs-

Gardner, C., Klazand, A., & Alhassan, S. (200, March 7). Comparison of the Atkins, Zone, Ornish, and LEARN Diets for Change in Weight and Related Risk Factors Among Overweight Premenopausal Women The A TO Z Weight Loss Study: A Randomized Trial. JAMA Network. https://jamanetwork.com/journals/jama/fullarticle/205916

How It Works. (n.d.). Atkins. https://www.atkins.com/how-it-works

Low Carb Diet Rules of Induction. (n.d.). Atkins. https://www.atkins.com/how-it-works/library/articles/the-rules-of-induction

Mandes, T. (2014, December 09). *The Difference Between Processed and Refined Foods*. Trisha Mandes. http://www.trishamandes.com/blog/2014/12/8/the-difference-between-processed-and-refined-foods

Metcalfe, R. (2019, March 20). *Even light physical activity has health benefits – new research*. The Conversation. https://theconversation.com/even-light-physical-activity-has-health-benefits-new-research-113700

Nutrition 101. (n.d.). Build Healthy Kids. http://www.buildhealthykids.com/basics.html

Scott, J. (2020, September 12). *What You Can Drink on the Atkins Diet*. Verywell Fit. https://www.verywellfit.com/what-you-can-drink-during-induction-on-the-atkins-diet-3496207#:

Warburton, D., Nicol, C., & Bredin, S. (2006, March 14). *Health benefits of physical activity: the evidence*. NCBI. https://www.ncbi.nlm.nih.gov/pmc/articles/PMC1402378/

What are Net Carbs? How to Calculate Net Carbs. (n.d.). Atkins. https://www.atkins.com/how-it-works/library/articles/what-are-net-carbs

IMAGE REFERENCES

Congerdesign. (2017, November 17). *Pumpkin Soup* [Photograph]. Pixabay. https://pixabay.com/photos/pumpkin-soup-soup-2972858/

Free-Photos. (2015, September 11). *Dinner* [Photograph]. https://pixabay.com/photos/meal-food-dinner-lunch-restaurant-918639/

J. (2017, December 3). *Sprouts, avocado, berries, lettuce, and nut board* [Photograph]. https://pixabay.com/photos/broccoli-sprouts-super-food-1977732/

Kerdkanno, S. (2015, August 28). *Baking* [Photograph]. https://pixabay.com/photos/background-baker-baking-cooking-906135/

Kulesza, M. (2018, May 15). *Don't Give Up* [Photograph]. https://pixabay.com/photos/don-t-give-up-motivation-3403779/

PhotoMix-Company. (2016, May 27). *Strawberry Smoothie* [Photograph]. https://pixabay.com/photos/strawberry-smoothie-kefir-the-drink-1418212/

Reche, D. (2020, June 22). *Walking/Running* [Photograph]. https://pixabay.com/photos/running-sport-race-athlete-hall-4782721/

StockSnap. (2017, July 31). *Yoga/Pilates* [Photograph]. https://pixabay.com/photos/people-woman-yoga-meditation-2562357/

Tuso, J. (n.d.). *Nutritional Update for Physicians: Plant-Based Diets.* NCBI. https://www.ncbi.nlm.nih.gov/pmc/articles/PMC3662288/

Vegan Liftz. (2019, May 27). *Meal Plan* [Photograph]. https://pixabay.com/photos/meal-plan-diet-plan-eating-healthy-4232109/

Wellington, J. (2018, March 11). *Basket of brown eggs.* https://pixabay.com/photos/brown-eggs-breakfast-nutrition-food-3217675/